MIRACLES
IN
MINUTES

A doctor and patient's guide
to alleviating the most
pains almost immediately

JOSEPH P. WOOD, D.C.

C O N T E N T S

ACKNOWLEDGMENTS

I would like to thank my family for allowing me the time to grow and explore many new things. I recognize that they are miracles in my life, and I thank them for their encouragement, support, and steadfastness.

I would like to thank all of my patients who were willing to trust me, work with me, and help me find answers to challenging and difficult cases. By working together, we found solutions not only for you, but for others also.

INTRODUCTION

Miracles in Minutes was written to share the protocols I developed to alleviate pain for many conditions often instantly. To do this, the reader (Doctor or Patient) will learn how to look at a problem with a 'new set of eyes.' You will learn that what you believe as the source of the problem is often not the source, or pain generator.

Most patients and doctors have already spent enormous amounts of time and money on the area that hurts, yet the patient still has pain, or the pain has changed very little. I concluded that the area being treated is frequently not the problem because if it were, the problem would have been resolved with treatment.

I started looking in different areas of the body to find the source of the patient's problem and soon developed protocols that alleviated pain, often in just minutes. I starting to find ways to achieve instant relief for certain conditions and this lead me to explore the concept further. After six years of exploration, I wrote *Miracles in Minutes* to share what I have learned.

The information in this book has proven to be effective for about 85 percent of the most common complaints presented by patients in pain. While this book is not written to provide a cure, it opens a doorway to help a patient who is struggling with pain. The patient can get relief quickly and safely, in many instances, if the patient follows the protocols outlined in this book.

Some people are looking for "proof" that this stuff works. When I wrote this book I only had clinical experience. After completion of the initial framework of the book I later came across the works of Dr. Vladamir Janda, M.D., who wrote about the same things I observed clinically. He identifies a few patterns that he calls: *Lower Cross Syndrome*, *Upper Cross Syndrome*, and *Layered Syndrome*. While I have never been a student of Dr. Janda, I was gratified to discover an empirical explanation for why this method is so effective.

This book details a fast, effective way to eliminate pain by simply affecting neurology and reflexes. What has someone in pain is a reflex controlled by the brain. Once we understand why the reflex is occurring it can be shut off almost instantly when the right input is placed into the system (body).

This book is written not only for my colleagues, but also for the patient, personal trainers, Yoga instructors, Pilates instructors, athletic trainers and for people interested in finding relief.

Too often, debilitating pain ruins a patient's ability to enjoy life. *Miracles in Minutes* is a simplistic guide that provides a doctor or patient a series of stretches and exercises to apply to specific pain patterns. The goal is to provide relief faster and more effectively than medication. I hope you enjoy this powerful, yet simplistic method. I call: *Miracles in Minutes*.

"The doctor of the future will give no medicine, but will interest her or his patients in the care of the human frame, in a proper diet, and in the cause and prevention of disease."

~ *Thomas Edison (U.S. inventor, 1847-1931)*

CHAPTER ONE

DR. WOOD'S THREE COMMANDMENTS

Once upon a time there was a man named Christopher Columbus. At the time Columbus lived, everyone thought the world was flat -except him. He did not believe everything he was taught about the world. Instead, he explored new ideas. In doing so, Columbus discovered the New World.

Miracles in Minutes is the result of my finding a new world within the field of healthcare after years of clinical experience. It is a summary of the methods and techniques I have used to achieve fast and effective results for my patients for some of the simplest, to some of the most difficult problems I have treated. The person can expect a predictable outcome a majority of the time if he/she follows the rules and methods described in this book. Some cases will be more difficult than others, but what I offer are sound, simple, highly-effective principles that, if applied correctly, will alleviate most common musculoskeletal problems within minutes. My goal in writing this book is to provide the tools to *miraculously* alleviate a person's pain in as little as ten minutes.

You may be wondering what complex or new neurological terms you will learn. Hopefully, there will be none. The idea is to *simplify, simplify, and simplify*. I have spent years reading, learning, studying, and experimenting with various exercises and techniques. The system that I developed as a result is a combination of Yoga, core moves, Pilates, functional training, rehab techniques, posture exercises, and martial arts warm-ups in various combinations which proved to be effective in alleviating my patients' complaints.

I recognize patterns and systems and how they fit together. There are many experts in certain fields of study or techniques. I am not an expert. The only thing I am concerned with is achieving results. The question I ask is: Does it work or doesn't it? It is my belief that every discipline has something to offer, so I combined certain exercises with others, and in the process discovered a system that produces remarkable results.

In brief, this book will give you a simple, efficient way to detect and alleviate common musculoskeletal problems. But first, let me introduce you to my three commandments:

1. **Never create or reproduce the symptoms.**
2. **Always respect the Great Physician/Innate Intelligence.**
3. **Always use perfect form and technique.**

Before you learn the protocols, you must learn my three commandments. The commandments provide a framework to operate in for safety's sake.

Commandment number one, if broken, will cause big trouble every time. If a person is doing an exercise or stretch and he is experiencing joint pain or nerve pain and we continue even though "he innately knows" we should stop, we will cause a lot of trouble. He exclaims, "This exercise is hurting my shoulder!" That means CEASE now!

Helping someone is easy if one listens to the Great Physician/Innate intelligence. By the way, the Great Physician is not any doctor or therapist but a wisdom or inner voice that exists in the body that just "knows." Knows how to heal something, allow things to function properly, and seeks to do what is "best" for the body. This innate intelligence is sort of a program that runs outside our awareness and heals torn skin, broken bones, grows hair, etc. Its alarm voice is pain or tightness. And its "yes, please do this" voice is a sense of ease, relaxation, peace or a 'sigh'.

Pain, we could say, is a state of negative stress or distress. Our bodies operate wonderfully in a state of relaxation or peace. Pain, an alarmed voice from within, is a call for change of some sort and is exclaiming **P**ay **A**ttention **I**nside **N**ow! Something is wrong and needs to be addressed. We should not ignore it or cover it up.

Most of us can figure out that if "this" hurts then we should stop doing the "this". This could be golfing, racquetball picking up our children, or some other movement. Others do it anyway and find themselves in bad shape by ignoring the signals or communication.

The *Miracles in Minutes* System is looking for the Relief, or the thing to do which will help the body can heal itself. The "signs" of hitting the nail on the head are discussed later in this book, but it should be a state of ease and peace.

The 3rd commandment is to pay attention to the details of correct form and technique. To achieve the results of the *Miracles in Minutes* System, the three commandments must be adhered to.

Many doctors utilize techniques or exercises that follow a certain learned method. We try to match these methods with our patients' needs and many times this does not work. A lot of well-meaning people have devised approaches or recommend "things" that worked for them and their issue. This can lead to limited "solutions" and sometimes the "method" or form of care actually can make some people worse. Whatever the protocol, or method of care chosen for whichever condition, I always follow my 3 commandments.

Now let's review:

COMMANDMENT #1: NEVER REPRODUCE THE SYMPTOMS.

In this book are many suggestions to help someone. If a suggested exercise or stretch is increasing pain or creating joint pain or something is getting tingly then stop immediately. Every person is unique and what works for one person may not work for someone else. The real doctor is located within the patient and that innate intelligence, or Great Physician, knows exactly what is wrong and how to fix it. It is this same innate intelligence that secretes enzymes to digest food, reach sexual maturity, makes the heart beat perfectly, moves the eyes around etc. Innate is that *little inner voice* that informs a person, for example, that she is having a heart attack and should go to the ER immediately.

COMMANDMENT #2: ALWAYS RESPECT THE GREAT PHYSICIAN and INNATE INTELLIGENCE

Commandment number two requires you to defer to the Great Physician every time. ALWAYS RESPECT INNATE INTELLIGENCE. We *assume* we know and we need to be open-minded first before we dig into a mode of care. We need to do a little of the proposed care first to validate that the proposed method is effective for a particular person vs. a presupposition that it worked for "Mary, who had back pain" thus it will work for "Jane, who also has back pain."

The Great Physician has also designed the body to compensate for injury or illness, so that we continue to have primary function, but we do so in a dysfunctional way. Mary may compensate differently than Jane for an issue, yet both have "back pain."

Each individual is equipped with this inner voice that can help rectify an issue. To speak with the Great Physician/Inner Voice/Innate Intelligence, just communicate in a simple manner. Ask him to let you know if what you are doing is **making the issue worse** or if it is **making it better**. That is as simple as it gets.

I am also following _Pareto's Law_ or the 80/20 principle. We are looking for an exercise or stretch that produces an 80% result with a 20% effort, or maximum reward for minimal effort. The universe, business, and life offer the greatest rewards to those who adhere to Pareto's Law. We call it being _EFFECTIVE_ and being _EFFICIENT_.

The body is wired for effectiveness and efficiency. For example, we initiate jogging as our form of exercise. At first it is very challenging, but in time it becomes easier. The brain has found a way to make this exercise more effective and efficient.

COMMANDMENT #3: ALWAYS USE PERFECT FORM AND TECHNIQUE

The third commandment is very simple: _ALWAYS USE PERFECT FORM AND TECHNIQUE_. The subtle details in the instructions are what make many of the stretches and exercises effective. If things aren't working out then reread the instructions of the exercise. Maybe the technique is a little off in applying the exercise?

If things still are not working out then we are just "doing something" vs. keeping an eye on Pareto's law, very little effort and maximum result. We need to move on for when the appropriate stimulus is uploaded into the CNS (body/nervous system) it is like a key to a locked door... things just open up magically.

5

One does NOT have to "do" all the exercises suggested. We are not seeing "how many things" we can do but what is the least we can do, and produce the greatest results… the *Miracle*.

When a patient suffers from severe conditions and pain patterns, I try to find **two movement patterns** the patient can do without causing himself pain. If I find two patterns that work effectively on someone who is in severe pain, then I have the patient repeat those two exercises. Once the patient's pain subsides the best thing to do is, LEAVE IT ALONE. Allow the body to just calm down.

For example, someone has severe back pain, a "10/10" (pure agony.) The pain then drops to a "5/10" then LEAVE IT ALONE.

This book is more like rescuing a drowning swimmer rather than giving swimming lessons. If we follow this simple method correctly and adhere to my three commandments, then miracles will happen—often within minutes.

I cannot promise that some unexpected things will not occur as one applies the principles in this book. There is no way for me to prepare a person for every possibility. However, the system I developed is designed to address any unexpected situations safely and effectively. Again, just follow my three commandments:

1. **Do not reproduce or increase the pain.**
2. **Trust the wisdom of the body or Innate Intelligence.**
3. **Use good form and technique.**

Keep it simple. Do a little bit, and if it helps then… "ok" do a little more. If the pain goes up then STOP immediately. By doing just a little bit, **meaning a few seconds of the exercise or stretch**, we can stay in a sort of safety-zone while exploring a possible solution, or in this case… the *Miracle in Minutes*.

CHAPTER TWO

UNDERSTANDING THE BLUEPRINT

We understand anatomy and the way the body operates. We evaluate and study the details in the individual systems. Let's apply what we already know to some simple examples.

Let us think of a body like a house. Each house is built with a specific blueprint; any deviation from the design compromises the structural integrity of the house. Every house has footers, a foundation, support beams, and load-bearing walls. Of course, the house has electrical wiring, plumbing, and even a computer system to monitor the functioning of all of the systems of the house. The footers of a house secure its foundation; the foundation is what transfers the weight of the house onto the ground below it, much like our feet transfer our weight onto the ground. Obviously, the foundation is the most critical structural component. Similarly, the low back forms the foundation of our bodies.

The bones and muscles are the support structure. When bones meet they connect, and we call them joints. Joints can have different abilities. Some joints hinge like a door. The knee is a hinge joint. It only likes to bend one way which is forward and back.

Other joints allow the body to rotate and spin like the wrist, ankles, hips and shoulders. The mid back likes to rotate but the low back does not.

If we only had hinge joints we would move like Frankenstein but the wonderful design of the body enables an infinitum of movements and activity.

If the body becomes misaligned and/or suffers an injury, we have to compensate to continue to move. A spinning joint like the ankle may lose the ability to spin so now the knee spins. Knees do not like to spin; they like to hinge or move forward and back. But since we need to move, the body will enable the knee to do some additional things to allow movement.

The body is designed to survive; thus if we suffered an injury in battle we could still limp, crawl, hop and do whatever to flee the scene to survive. But once the battle is over, we need to see if the body returned to its normal alignment and operating function.

When the body is beginning to run out of compensating strategies, we experience pain. The knee may hurt, but it could be due to an ankle that stopped functioning properly. Pain calls out to restore the alignment and function. In this case we would want to restore the function to the ankle. Pain says "we have lost our effectiveness and efficiency," please address this issue now.

If these misalignments are not addressed, a person will learn to adapt to the new faulty alignment(s) and every time the body moves, it keeps twisting up more and more. Slowly over time, tension builds; we might call it stress, pain(s) or things "getting on our nerves." The healthy functioning of every system in our bodies hinges on proper structural alignment. When any part of the body deviates from its proper alignment, it elicits a signal that something is wrong. We call these signals "symptoms" but the question we might ask is… what is CAUSING the symptoms?

Most care or treatment is focused on the symptom(s) and thus many a person never really resolves the issue, so the brain works around the problem and the pain returns at a later date or "somewhere else."

Patient: "My ankle is better but now my knee hurts."

Doctor: "Oh, you must have a knee problem now. What did you do?"

Doesn't it begin to look like a dog chasing his tail? Are we moving from one pain to the next with the next form of treatment for the knee now? Or was it never an "ankle issue" to begin with and the ankle merely "hurt" or was painful? Care ensued to "fix" or "cover up" the ankle pain signals and now the body compensated to alleviate the pain in the ankle by SHOVING the stress into the knee.

For some the brain can weight shift in a way to have one "believe" the issue is resolved. How do we know the issue is resolved by most people's standards? The answer: One has no pain at the present moment.

Pain is the last thing to appear and the first thing to disappear. One has to be very dysfunctional to have pain. The CNS (central nervous system) can "adapt" to some really weird things that ARE NOT helpful such as smoking, for example Smoking is NOT per se' healthy, yet the body can adapt to smoking and NOT have any pain whatsoever.

Person: "It doesn't hurt to smoke. My lungs don't hurt. I am good to go."

Dr.: "How about we check your tidal volume of oxygen getting into your lungs which is a FUNCTION."

9

One has to lose ALMOST full capacity of the FUNCTION of the lungs to have "lung pain." Then it might be too late, but there will be early symptoms such as coughing or bronchitis or other frequent lung issues and even blue finger nails.

THE ABSENCE OF PAIN IS <u>NOT</u> AN INDICATOR OF HEALTH!

Is the body FUNCTIONING properly?

Function might be predicated on or built upon "structure" first. And to build a structure, one would follow a "blueprint".

If we understand the blueprint and how the body is designed to function then we can interface better and thus see *Miracles in Minutes.*

The structure is a balanced configuration of the ankle, knee, hip and shoulder, lined up like two side-by-side studs in a wall in the up/down front view. Then the shoulders, hips, knees and ankles should be lined up with the horizon as well. The feet should point directly ahead. It is a system of 90 degree angles much like the way our homes are constructed.

The 90 degree angles create lift and we have a very "top heavy" structure with a "high" center of gravity. The alignment of the joints enables the body to have fluid movement and incredible infinite abilities: football to ballet, to playing a piano, or rock climbing.

To have ALL the potential to do almost anything we want to do, the body is set up as a system of stable and mobile joints as discussed by Gray Cook, PT and Mike Boyle. The "stable/mobile theory" or the "joint by joint" theory:

- **A stable foot.**
- **A mobile ankle.**

- **A stable knee.**
- **A mobile hip.**
- **A stable low back.**
- **A mobile mid back.**
- **A stable shoulder blade.**
- **A mobile shoulder/arm.**

This system of stable and mobile joints allows for human movement. When a mobile joint stops moving, like an ankle, the body gets mobility or movement from a joint that does not like to move, such as the low back or knee.

Man is designed to be bipedal, or walk upright on two legs. If we think about it, this is a miraculous balancing act. Over 120 bones and 600 muscles have to work in concert to lift us up, and then move us around. Part of the miracle is the design and the shape of our spine which looks like a spring. The brain coordinates the "stable/mobile" joint system to lift the body upright balanced on two legs. There is a specific system in the body for posture called the PVV system or *Proprioception Visual Vestibular*

Proprioception: This means the brain knows ALL the body at any time. The brain knows the condition and ability of each joint, muscle, tendon, and has the capability to control the joint. It knows how well the heart and stomach, etc are doing. It knows **ALL** the body at any time. The brain is the commander or CEO of this organism.

Think of *proprioception* as the body parts telling the brain how well they are functioning.

If we "sprain" our ankle the brain is quickly aware and we might limp or hop to prevent further damage. The *proprioceptive* system told the brain there was a problem and the brain took a corrective course of action to ensure the "wellbeing" of the person. The pain

11

in the ankle is there to PREVENT the person from damaging the joint further.

Visual: The eyes help us to balance ourselves but we still have two other systems as backups. People who are blind can still walk. If there is a loss or "dysfunction" in part of the body, other parts make up for the loss. Some people become *visual dominant*.

An example of visual dominancy is an elderly person who uses his eyes to maintain balance. The person's eyes typically stare at his feet to prevent a fall.

Vestibular: This is related to the ear. We all are aware of people who have a really bad inner ear infection and then develop severe dizziness, losing the ability to stand and move around. Inside the ear is something called the *cochlea* which is a structure of three tubes of fluid containing hairs. As we move, the fluid moves and touches the hairs providing information on where our body is located in space and if we are falling or losing our balance.

The nervous system can be thought of as system of messages. When something causes the nerve to fire, a message is sent in response. Messages go to the brain, and messages come from the brain to the area affected. This occurs throughout the body. The PVV system is just one part of the nervous system.

Misalignment of joints can affect posture, which can have very dramatic effects on health. There is NOT a lot of room in the body to be losing space or suffering *cave-ins*.

Think of it this way... If one of the support walls in one's family-room slides out of place, the wall it supports could collapse or move.

A loss of structural alignment affects the posture of the body. As the following studies found:

12

Older People with weak posture had a 1.44x greater mortality rate:

Study of 1,353 osteoporosis patients:

- Posture was assessed as Normal or Hyperkyphotic (forward head). Hyperkyphotic was defined as requiring more than a 1.7 cm head support hold head level.
- **People with hyperkyphotic (Forward head) posture had a 1.44x greater mortality over the next 4.2 years.**

D. Kado, MD, Huang, DrPH, A. Karlamangla, MD, PhD etc. Journal of the American Geriatrics Society, Volume 52 issue 10, p 1662 –10/2004

Bad posture could raise blood pressure:

There is a direct neural connection between neck muscles and nucleus tractus solitarius (NTS – a part of the brainstem which plays a crucial role in regulating heart rate and blood pressure.)

Study author: I.J. Edwards

This study could explain elevated BP and heart rate with neck injuries like whiplash or ergonomic activities like hunched over a computer all day.

The Journal of Neuroscience, DOI: 10.1523/neurosci.0638-07.2007

"Forward Head Posture leads to long term muscle strain, disc herniation, arthritis... "

Mayo Clinic, November 3rd, 2000

Deviations in the body's center of gravity (read: poor posture)... have resulted in intestinal problems, hemorrhoid, varicose veins, osteoporo-

13

sis, hip and foot deformities, POOR HEALTH, DECREASED QUALITY OF LIFE, and a SHORTENED LIFE SPAN. [my emphasis added].

Journal of the American Medical Association, Volume 165(7), pages 843-846

"For every inch of forward head posture, it can increase the weight of the head on the spine by an additional 10 pounds."

Dr. Kapandji, Physiology of Joints -- Volume 3

These studies clearly show a clinical relationship between health issues and body alignment. By becoming a little more educated about joints, muscles, tendons, tissues and the nervous system, we can possibly have dramatic health benefits with little effort.

The PVV system may sound complicated, or one may wonder how posture and alignment could cause something as far reaching as anxiety, depression or "dementia".

To understand this a little more in relation to the PVV system I will use an airplane as an example. A pilot uses a gyroscope to maintain his orientation in space, thereby establishing the location of the horizon. If a pilot loses track of the horizon, he could lose his bearings and crash. The instrumentation panel provides all the information needed to the pilot to still fly in darkness and all kinds of weather.

The body is wonderfully made to include gyroscope-like structures in our ears known as *cochlea* that orient our bodies to keep us from falling. When our head moves forward and in front of the shoulders, the body's gyroscopes tell the brain that the body is falling. However, the eye tells the brain that the body is not falling.

Close your eyes and look down. What sensation are you experiencing?

In theory this single postural misalignment could cause a myriad of "symptoms" such as confusion, dizziness, and anxiety because the brain is receiving diametrically opposed pieces of information.

Vestibular/cochlea to brain: "You are falling."

Eye: "No, you are not."

Vestibular/cochlea: "Yes, you are."

Eye: "No, you are not."

Brain: "Guys, get your act together! I am confused."

Are we falling or not? On a subconscious level, these bits of information are confusing the brain, which must continually adjust more than 600 muscles to keep the body upright. Can you see how this could cause a distraction to the brain resulting in the loss of concentration, which in turn creates forgetfulness and anxiety?

Is this a possible reason why elderly people become forgetful? What is more important; our conversations, remembering to get "bread" or falling? To the brain a fall striking one's head is MORE IMPORTANT to survival. For if the brain is seriously damaged then life ends rather quickly. So preventing a head injury needs ALL of our attention inwardly. The outward conversations and needs are not relevant at this time.

Daughter: "Dad is becoming very forgetful."

Is Dad forgetful or has attention shifted to discerning the postural balance to walk and stand? Dad has to *think* about how to balance vs. it occurring automatically.

We are not designed to think about balancing, for it should be automatic. We should not have to think about how to get off the

15

floor, out of a chair or make our heart beat. These are handled for us by the innate wisdom of the CNS or brain, via reflexes.

As people get older and you place them on the floor, they have to wait and think about how to get up. The pop or spring is not there anymore. Most people simply just believe that age is the reason why. What does the POSTURE look like on people who do not move well?

What does the POSTURE look like of an Olympic track and field athlete? I have not seen a hot-shot Olympian with poor posture have you? Just maybe the ALIGNMENT can influence the ability? And "posture" is merely a window into how well the CNS is functioning.

If the body loses the structural alignment the system has to work harder to do simple tasks. This leads to fatigue from the inefficiency. The body is working hard and the signal that it has *had enough* is pain, or some other symptoms.

The solution that I came to was; let's understand the design and the function of the body and then "how to" safely interact with the body to allow the healing and rejuvenation to naturally take place. The body is designed to heal and rejuvenate itself constantly. But if there is something interfering with the natural process of rejuvenation and healing, the healing cannot take effect.

We need to take a "corrective course" of action to restore the function and thus HEALTH returns. *Miracles in Minutes* is the "outside the box" exploration of a return to health. The commandments and Pareto's Law are the guides I use to explore part of the blueprint and design of the body that can keep one on the "narrow road" destination to our goal of optimum health.

THE DESIGN

Part of alignment is a system of stabilizing muscles. These muscles are very tiny and are designed to contract just enough to keep the spine and joints in place. The *rotator cuff* is a stabilizing muscle of the shoulder.

In the spine are three small muscle groups that allow front to back, side to side and rotational movement.

The stabilizing system should fire first, and then BIG muscles called *prime movers* fire next. A prime mover includes the deltoid or shoulder muscle, the quad or thigh, and the hamstring. Prime movers generate lots of power but have limited capacity for continued work at maximum effort.

When an injury occurs or high stress is placed on the body, the stabilizers shut down and the prime movers take over the job of stabilizing. The prime mover is way too powerful for the job, but the body can do anything it needs to continue movement.

Prime movers like to contract and relax. The bicep can only do so many repetitions in the gym before it is burnt out and won't contract anymore. The brain can call upon the bicep to assist in stabilizing the shoulder if need be. The problem is that the bicep is designed to contract and relax, whereas stabilizers are designed to be continuously at work; like our heart.

If a prime mover is recruited to be a stabilizer for a long time the muscle begins to change its function. This could go on for years, and now our grand mom cannot raise her arms over her head. The muscles that should move the shoulder have become stabilizers, and stabilizers do not like to move. So our grandmother suffers in pain, is stiff, and cannot move like she wants.

17

The muscles that should move grand mom's shoulder have been recruited to balance the body. If a person loses her balance the arms "whip out" to regain the balance. The arms/shoulders are now acting as stabilizers to keep the body upright. The solution should have been realized a LONG TIME AGO to restore the function and balance vs. keep on suffering with an injury.

Our "ego" and "willpower" can get us into trouble. We negate the internal communication of: "Houston, we have a problem." And if Mrs. Houston doesn't address this problem, her arm will soon be like… grand mom's.

Yet, our "will" and "ego" can keep us going. The brain can figure out a way to *work around the issue* but eventually the issue catches up with us. Old age does not have to be a life of pain. How the system lost its design, or became unstable is not an exact science; and neither is medicine, physical therapy, or chiropractic. As healthcare providers we do our best, but there is much to learn.

Pain is not well-understood, but it is thought to be tied into the limbic system which is our emotional system, and the specific emotion of fear. When we are afraid we "tighten up" to protect ourselves. For some reason a prime mover is told to stay on the job of stabilizing a joint, while still performing its other activities.

The *Miracles in Minutes System* is designed to allow the prime mover to take a break and reveal or "wake up" the stabilizing muscles. Once the body goes back to the original design specifications, the vigor and vitality of our youth reappears. It was not lost but covered over with ineffective movements and layers of protection from a previous injury/fear response. That is my *best guess* at what might be occurring.

Proper alignment and a well-functioning nervous system is what allows children to develop the ability to walk and run with agility, strength, and energy. Watch a toddler run. A toddler can run all day and never get tired or out of breath. They do not push with their muscles but are pulled up, almost effortlessly. This is why they skip and jump. A toddler moves using reflexes vs. pushing or exerting muscular effort.

The difference between the two is night and day. Reflexes vs. "exertion" can be felt in the demonstration below:

Do this:

Place your hand on your chest. Now lift your index finger. Now as hard as you can, smash your finger into your chest. Keep lifting the finger and then as hard as you physically can, have the finger strike the chest over and over for about 12 seconds. Getting tired yet?

Now do this: Place hand in the same position with all the fingers resting on the chest, but now take your other hand and stretch your finger back and stay relaxed. Now pull it back kind of far and then let it go. BAM! How much more POWER was that? How much effort?

A lot more power and almost zero effort by just pulling the finger back. Reflex movement is much more efficient than mere muscular exertion. Making use of the GTR or *golgi tendon reflex* to move enables more natural lifting and movement patterns. Thus kids spring, skip and bounce because they are moving differently than most adults and using different methods.

The "good news" is that the childlike qualities of movement and joy are still there but just covered over with ineffective movement strategies. Ineffective movement strategies fatigue the nervous system and wear us down. We might call it, *burnout* or pain.

19

When the body is out of alignment we must choose a strategy of muscular effort to move like the finger demonstration above.

Thus the "design" of the body or structural alignment is what allows the reflex movement. Evaluating posture against the "blueprint" can help us understand a possible solution or "miracle" for the pain a person is experiencing.

Just having a person stand can provide a lot of information about how well the nervous system is functioning and how balanced structurally a person is.

Some people stand with one foot in front of the other. People's head cock to the side. One shoulder is higher than the other, and feet point out vs. straight ahead.

All we know is this: The body is not functioning optimally if the normal alignment is not presenting in front of us. t simply reverts back to the scientific studies that say posture can affect many things and cause all kinds of symptoms. We are just aware that the nervous system is not operating efficiently and some "corrective course" of action is warranted.

The normal side posture view should reveal the ankle, knee, hip, and shoulder in perfect linear alignment with the ear falling in line with the shoulder. Upon walking, the knee should track or fall directly over the ankle and the foot should point directly forward.

It should NOT be a forced thing. A person should walk normal and just observe the way he or she stands and walks. As noted earlier, these are automatic responses from the brain. We should not have to *think* about walking normally; it should just happen naturally.

Our first "natural response" to when we observe something out of place or not functioning properly is to "fix it." So a person observes someone who walks "funny" and then we recommend a series of exercises or braces, or treatments to "make" it work right.

The brain did not forget "how to" have things work properly. Something is interfering with "normal operations" of function. A joint may be out of place, or a muscle is contracting abnormally and we need to learn to relax it by a stretch or some activity.

The body's design is incredible, intelligent, and maybe beyond our full comprehension much like the universe. But we can observe the architecture and observe some laws of physics to interact with the wisdom/innate intelligence that enables our body parts to function appropriately.

The unique thing about this design is that from a mechanical view, the joints are positioned to be on a perfect pivot. A perfect pivot occurs when a structure is perfectly balanced and requires little motion or effort to move it. This phenomenon is illustrated in several ways, one of which is the story of the *Coral Castle*, which tells how a man hung a six-ton door on a perfect pivot. The door was so easy to open that a two year old could open it by pushing her fingertip against the door. A perfect pivot eliminates friction or resistance, which prevents wear and tear on the hinge. On a perfect pivot a six-ton door is weightless!

Our joints are not designed to wear out in our 30's or 40's but to last a lifetime. On a perfect pivot the joints would remain relatively healthy forever, theoretically. Most people have never felt the "optimum health effect" from a properly functioning body.

Several wonderful things occur when our bodies are working properly and our joints are acting as perfect pivots. First, the patient instantly feels **taller**. Secondly, he feels **lighter**. Thirdly, he will be **very happy** and feel **ethereal**. Finally, he will feel like he has **springs for legs** and his **energy will increase**. This is how we are

21

meant to feel when the wonderful machine we have been given is operating properly.

How and why do all these things occur? When the muscles let go, the body lengthens and the loss of resistance causes movement to occur with much less effort. Remember, you always have to apply more work or energy against resistance. Additionally, we took pressure off of the nervous system. If the spinal muscles are compressing then we are narrowing the holes between the backbones where nerves travel to control a certain part of the body. When the spinal muscles are compressed or stretched, the nerves are pinched, or irritated. Chiropractors call this a *subluxation*; meaning, bones have lost their normal position/alignment and the communication between the brain and end organ (muscle, joint, stomach, pancreas, etc.) is interrupted to some degree.

According to *Gray's Anatomy,* 29th edition page 4; "The nervous system controls and coordinates ALL structures and functions of the human body." It is easy to understand this concept if you know someone who has nerve damage. The area of the body that the nerve controls no longer works properly. The connection between brain and effected part is interrupted, and the greater the interruption the greater the malfunction, e.g. "I can't raise my arm." or a lesser degree "I can't open jars anymore." Or, "I drop things out my hands."

Innately or intuitively we are always doing things to get ourselves back into proper alignment. We will see people doing all kinds of "weird" stretches, wiggling, shifting in their chairs, etc. They stop wiggling and stretching when the alignment happens. Until they get back into normal alignment the person seems agitated, irritable, cranky, short-tempered, in pain or discomfort, lethargic, moody, or stops doing things. All of these are signs of stress to the nervous system.

When the spinal muscles are not compressed and the body is in optimum alignment, the pressure on the nervous system is relieved. The patient now feels free and liberated which is a powerful feeling. It is the best high of all, and is known as *Optimum Health*.

The nervous system, which handles ALL of our daily functions, needs a way to speak to us when it is challenged in taking care of us. That voice is symptoms, and the symptoms indicate an issue with function and/or structure and a problem with the Creator's original design.

Pain tells us something is wrong and that is all it means. Just because the "low back hurts" does not automatically mean that the low back is the issue or cause. If stretching the calf alleviated the pain in less than 20 seconds, what do we make of that?

The "low back" is under stress, but something else in the perfect-pivot design is causing excessive loading on the back. Sure the disc may have herniated, but why? We can see the herniated disc on the MRI, but this does not tell us the cause of herniation.

Some might say, "I picked up something heavy." Heavy is relative, and we are designed to do those type of activities. But if the body lost its LEVERAGE points to lift and the back was OVERSTRESSED due to a loss of structure and function, then sure... the RESULT could be a low back disc-herniation.

If the back is under a continuous cycle of loading and does not get to relax, then the back will surely fail. As noted above, if we look at the nature of the universe we can understand things better. The body likes to move in cycles. The heart contracts and then it relaxes. Air comes in and air goes out which is mediated by the diaphragm; the *breathing* muscle. Another way of observing this is ON and then OFF. On is contract, and off is relax.

23

If the body gets stuck in phase, or is always "on", then it does not get to relax in order to rejuvenate. Tissue failure will occur, as in this case, a back injury. The pain and injury now have the person "shut down", or being forced to relax and take it easy. But if we discovered the CAUSE and what is not functioning, then a *Miracle in Minutes* can be achieved.

So far we have discovered:

1. **Things need to *line up*, creating perfect pivots, allowing reflex movement.**
2. **Things need to *function* in an optimum *cycle* of turning on and off at the appropriate times. These on/off cycles happen at an unconscious level, and faster than we can think, or process information consciously.**

Let's use a little more common sense to understand two more laws of physics: *Potential energy*, which is the energy that is stored in an object or system, and *kinetic energy*, which is the energy of motion. Potential energy is converted into Kinetic energy.

For example, when we pull a slingshot back, the bands become tight (potential energy). When we let go of the bands, the rock goes flying (kinetic energy). Similarly, when a patient's muscles are tight, we know his potential is not being released -physically or mentally. As the person moves, more tension is loaded onto the muscles. If this pattern continues, the body will send pain signals so the muscles do not rupture, break, or cause damage to a joint.

Creating a sensation of pain is often the way the body protects itself from injury. When the tension is released, the body feels better, moves better, and energy returns rather than drains away.

If the muscle cannot turn off, then the muscle is stuck in the "on" phase. The body cannot take a break to restore itself, and anything left on too long will breakdown. We are looking for the "relief valve" using the information provided so far.

We are going to use Pareto's Law, or the 80/20 Principle, when working with the design. We are going to be OPEN to anything and everything. We are going to forgo the myopic... "My back hurts," and the conclusion that one has a back problem.

Now that we have covered the basics of alignment, we need to understand mechanical motion. Surprisingly, we rarely stand on two feet. Most of the time, we are balancing on one foot. Our *modus operandi* for basic movement, as humans, is walking. To walk, one foot must be on the ground while the other must leave it to take a step forward. This requires quite a bit of balance. Most of us take it for granted, walking that is. But if we observe people walk, we can see very few actually move with grace, or optimum movement.

Try this: Stand on one leg. Now close your eyes. Can you do this for 30 seconds? Is your foot still or is it wobbling?

This posture is part of the "stance" phase for walking. Instability here reveals a lot about total health and determines whether a person should begin a walking program. The people who cannot balance here will only get better at walking poorly.

What we typically see are "waddles", hip swinging, pelvic thrusting, forward leans, backward leans, knock knees, bowed legs, feet draggers, and shufflers, etc.

The body is designed to move gracefully and fluidly. Our bodies are mainly made of water so the body should move like water; freely and fluidly.

If the body is out of alignment and not functioning properly, many a fitness routine may do more harm than good. A person

25

who cannot fully move his shoulder perhaps should not be lifting weights.

It is true one can have an OUTWARD appearance of "health" via development of the musculature, but that does not mean the system is "healthy" or functioning properly.

The CNS or Brain does not care how well our "ego muscles" look. It cares about movement, which from the hardwired survival aspect would allow us to get the basics:

1. **Air**
2. **Food**
3. **Water**
4. **Shelter**

If an individual is experiencing pain while walking it is a indicator of some serious issues with the overall health of the body. Walking is one of the best exercises for us, but for some walking can reinforce a faulty movement pattern. Someone who "waddles" when he walks will just "waddle" more on the treadmill.

What appears or sounds like a "good idea", neurologically and orthopedically may not be. Walking is NOT bad for us, but the way the person is walking or moving may be. Is the person's body lined up properly? Can the person move the joints and control the joints? If not, then why not? What is interfering with normal motion?

By understanding the body's design, function, and on and off cycles or what is normal, we can begin to understand how to help someone. We will be open to ANYTHING and assume nothing. Whatever enables normal walking or movement with a 20% effort and an 80% result is the method of choice and the *Miracles in Minutes* philosophy.

To me, this makes more sense in evaluating patients from a health perspective. I observe postural alignment and movements to help me understand what is malfunctioning, vs. looking at images like x-rays or MRIs.

MRI and x-ray are two dimensional; a living person who is interacting in my office is three dimensional. Now I can observe him in real-time and spot problems, causes, and find solutions.

Most patients don't come into the office complaining about their x-ray or MRI. They come in complaining about not being able to move or DO THINGS because of pain or inability. So why not evaluate movement to begin with? And before movement occurs we have basic posture and structural alignment.

CHAPTER THREE

PATIENT HISTORY AND EVALUATION

In today's modern world of Magnetic Resonance Imaging (MRI), Computerized Axial Tomography (CAT or CT scan) and other complex imaging systems, we often fail to pay close attention to what our patients are telling us because we rely on technology to reveal the patient's problem.

I am NOT saying that an X-ray or MRI does not give relevant information. These tools are very necessary for certain issues. However, from a cost perspective and from a regular exam process of health these tools become prohibitive. Yet we can evaluate posture and movement daily, without being exposed to radiation or fees.

It is imperative to take a complete history and perform a comprehensive evaluation when we first meet and examine the patient. We need to remember the real doctor is located within the patient; and that innate intelligence, or Great Physician, knows exactly what is wrong and how to fix it.

For any treatment to be successful, it is necessary to first establish a good line of communication; to do that, we need to establish rapport so that the patient feels comfortable and relaxed. Relaxation allows the parasympathetic nervous system a greater influence. As noted earlier, having many pain cycles is due to a sympathetic overload or "stress."

When the mind is agitated or a fear response is elicited, the *prefrontal cortex*, which is the smartest part of our brain in a sense is sort of shut down. Instead the amygdala, a very primitive part of the brain, kicks in and kind of begins running a loop of "what if's" or doubt and fear responses.

As the person relaxes, the pain loop cycle can now be let go and the body can heal itself. We need a new set of "eyes" to look at the current issue. Rapport, trust and relaxation will allow greater lines of communication with innate intelligence or the "Great Physician," or one could say the *prefrontal cortex*.

A patient cannot communicate what is going on if they are emotionally on edge. I often enter the exam room with a big smile and ask, "How are you doing?" Surprisingly, many people say, "Pretty good." Usually at that point I will exclaim, "If you were doing well you probably wouldn't be here!" Most people laugh, and that casual moment sets the tone for obtaining a good history.

The first thing we need to address is the patient's chief complaint, including the restrictions and limitations she is experiencing due to the complaint. We also need to quantify the complaint with a Visual Analog Scale (VAS scale) of 0-10; 10 being the highest level of pain, e.g., "I am dying," or in "complete agony."

VAS

0 1 2 3 4 5 6 7 8 9 10

0= no pain
5= moderate, and is creating some limitations in the ability to do things.
10= worst possible pain imaginable.

If you are a patient reading this, let me explain this in more detail. Doesn't it make sense to quantify our analysis via a number for one's pain-level and then later use that number to see if what the doctor is doing is helping? The **initial number is a baseline** to be used for determining the proper care path that is safe and effective.

For example, a patient says on the VAS, "I experience pain at #6/10 while standing." The doctor or "you", the patient, do some movement to see if the pain is going up or if "you", the patient, is moving better.

Let's suppose we start using the suggested exercises and stretches in this book, and as a result the pain goes to a #8/10. Then, it definitely means DON'T DO IT! Stop... now. The exercises and stretches in this book are **SUGGESTIONS** to what typically works for a certain issue. If something is not working then stop.

Now if the doctor is doing something and the pain is lessening, for instance a patient was a 6/10 and now they are a 1/10; then we just found out what we need to do. The VAS helps guide the doctor and the patient in a corrective course of action.

Once we find the "magic bullet" the FEAR of the issue is gone. The person now has a tool to help himself. To find the tool we must stay open to anything vs. the narrow-minded view of, "I have neck pain, so I must need a neck stretch or treatment." If stretching the calf for "neck pain" creates 90% relief in less than 30 seconds, why work so hard attempting to get the neck to relax or "loosen up"?

Here is the crux: We have been trained to be one-track minded, and assume the neck pain means a "neck problem." Neck pain merely means something is not functioning properly and most likely the neck is working double time.

Let's begin by remaining mentally neutral. No "preconceived thoughts," and merely listen to what the person is saying or what our nervous system is attempting to communicate to us; then begin our examination.

I listen very closely to what the patient says, and then I look for what is causing the complaint and the answer to the underlying question: why? At this point, I am totally aware of how the patient's body moves and holds itself upright. I observe **facial expressions, color and tension, as well as ease of movement, and breathing patterns during all forms of movement**.

These subtle clues are the *internal doctor* or our subconscious' way of telling us what is working. The "face" is the window to SEEING and OBSERVING the "truth", and leads us to the proper care selection.

For example, when I ask a patient to stand, I observe which foot hits the floor first. I also listen to her breathing. Is breathing labored? Does her face contort with pain? Can the patient move with ease? Is the patient stressed, anxious, or nervous? Look and listen!

You can gain much valuable information just by observing subtle body language. As treatment progresses, the patient's response to movement is one of the ways I determine whether the treatment is working. If it works, the patient's physical state will relax and motion improves. When we *hit the nail on the head*, the patient sighs or her eyebrows lift. Often, these subtle clues are followed by a verbal expression of satisfaction, such as, "Wow!" or "Ahh!"

Now let us see what else a simple standing test can reveal. Suppose an individual has right leg pain or right knee pain. I ask the patient to stand from a seated position, and he steps on the right foot first; and then uses his right side to support himself.

This simple action reveals that the cause of his problem will be found on the left side of his body. If he stands on the right leg or bears more weight on that side, and the complaint is on the right; I know that the right side of the body is doing all of the work.

Isn't it reasonable to assume that your leg would hurt if you continually used only one side of your body instead having the body *share the work* between the left and right sides?

Typically, the part of the body the patient complains about is the part that is doing all, or most of, the work! The real source of the problem typically, does not "complain". If the patient complains of neck pain, and we prescribe wonderful stretches for the neck, which result in marginal improvement; then the problem is most likely at the other end of the spine. If treatment is applied to the wrong part of the body, the treatment is not effective.

We do not want to treat symptoms. "My neck hurts, so treat the neck," is an example of treating symptoms. We do not want to *rush to judgment*, or limit the exam process yet. WHY does the neck hurt? WHY? We must stay in a system-analysis mode:

1. **Structural alignment and posture**
2. **Stable joints and mobile joints. What hurts is MOVING TOO MUCH, and the body has lost movement somewhere else.**
3. **How is the person breathing?: relaxed or stressed. With the belly, or neck and chest?**

If we simply treat the obvious symptom that hurts, then what typically happens is a marginal result.

At this point it is merely work for the sake of work. It is the experience of 80% effort and a 20% return. Sure things take time, such as weight-loss and emotional maturity; but movement was learned in early childhood. We are not learning something new, just uncovering the natural or authentic reflex movement we had as children.

This evaluation method and pattern of treatment deviates from most of what we have been taught. The problem with isolating the symptom is that sometimes we relegate the problem to "neck pain", instead of remembering that the neck is just one part of a complex structure. If the low back is unstable, which may not cause the patient pain; then it is possible the neck may be over compensating.

Most patients and doctors focus on the symptom instead of staying in a **system-analysis mode**. We need to establish ground-rules that include letting the patient know that he is the real "doctor." It is his body and his problem, and he knows a lot more about how to fix it than I do; because his body is telling him what to do. What I need from the patient is a line of communication with the Great Physician or subconscious telling me if what I am doing is improving the condition, or making it worse.

INPUT (stimulus) → OUTPUT (result) → GOOD keep doing (right stimulus), or BAD stop doing (wrong stimulus).

We are NOT attempting to "figure this out". We have a simple goal: We desire to move well, feel well, and move with ease and confidence.

We seek exercise or stretches that enable this to occur. Remember: pain is merely communication that something is not functioning properly. Pain actually has roots in fear, and the body has sort of a default fear response; which is the *fetal position*. In the nervous system, we call it the *hyper startle reflex*.

To see the hyper startle reflex in action; scare someone and watch what he does… Does he "duck and cover," or move into the fetal position?

The hyper startle reflex is a *fear state* or *protective state,* so the senses become heightened, and then the head will push forward to see the threat. It is impossible to identify and correct all of the patient's problems at once. Develop rapport, establish trust, and work on the problems one at a time. In just a few visits the patient will feel much better.

Some patients are nervous, and put their best foot forward; or put their "patient face" on during an examination. Patients ignore, deny, and rationalize their pains and problems; some patients are just poor communicators. But, for a person to achieve their desired outcome, or their desired health "destination"; he needs to know exactly where he is currently. If I want to go to New York City - the desired destination - then we need a reference point of the current location.

Is the person in Texas or Alaska, and desires to go to New York? We need to know where someone IS to reach the desired destination on a map and in health. Our clients, patients, and ourselves need to be honest with one another so that the GOAL can be achieved.

I have been in practice for 17 years, and no matter how many times I tell the patient I want to hear about his problems, I frequently learn more from my assistants, than I do from the Doctor-Patient conversation. Patients sometimes distort typical posture patterns, but as soon as they relax or act normal, the body reveals the problem. I strongly suggest that you **not** tell the patient you are evaluating his posture, because as soon as he knows this; he is likely to change his posture. If this is a self-exam then just stand "naturally" in a mirror and take a look. It is what it is. Now we have a reference point to begin from.

Other patients may be in so much pain that the only thing we can do is address the pain. We will have an extremely difficult time trying to correct a problem if a patient is in agony. When the pain subsides, we can begin to alleviate the problem; frequently faster than the patient has anticipated.

Whether we are in overhaul mode or pain-alleviation mode, **we need to identify the motion that improves the condition and all motion that causes the condition to worsen**.

Typically, but not always, the exact opposite motion of whatever motion makes a patient feel worse makes it better. For example, bending forward at the waist to "toe touch" makes the pain worse... STOP.

Now lean backwards. Did leaning backwards alleviate the pain? If so, then guess what we need to do? Lean backwards. Whatever the protocol you are using, always obey commandment number one: NEVER REPRODUCE THE SYMPTOMS.

During the administration of all range-of-motion and orthopedic tests, I observe and monitor all subtle, and subconscious body-language expressions. I make a mental note of any corrective motion that produces a **sigh of relief** or other acknowledgment of instant gratification because then I know what to do to alleviate the patient's pain and a "hint" at a very probable solution.

Two of the final aspects of the exam are balance/coordination, and something I call *life skills*. Life skills can be observed in doing the orthopedic and neurological evaluations. Basic life skills for a human body are rolling over, sitting up, standing from sitting (squats), getting on and off the floor from a prone position (push-ups), bending over to get something, and working above the head and evaluating whether the knees move toward each other when going from a sitting to a standing position.

Gray Cook, PT and many others, have contributed to something called *The Functional Movement Screen* or *FMS*. At the time of this writing I was looking to develop some metric to measure movement. I have since forgone that project since the task has been accomplished by Gray Cook, PT, CSCS.

Movement screening is an extremely valuable tool for understanding pain. Laymen should read Gray's book, *Athletic Body in Balance,* and for the professionals I recommend, *Movement.*

I use the speed of movement as an indicator for a corrective action as well as Gray's tools. Gray scores movement from a 0-3 scale on his movement screen. "0" indicates pain, and "3" is optimal.

The speed of movement after a corrective exercise or stretch can be a HUGE indicator of the appropriate action step. If a person moves faster and is more at ease then THAT is the stretch or exercise to do. Also did it follow Pareto's Law; or a small effort with a BIG result?

If the exercise or stretch causes the person to move slower, then we most likely do not want to repeat the exercise; although the person may "feel better".

The *feel good* sensation cannot be trusted. This goes against the popular mantra of society today, "if it feels good, do it."

The issue I have with "feel good" is this:

- Heroin makes people feel good.
- Cookies make people feel good.
- Spending money makes people feel good.
- Alcohol makes people feel good.
- Amphetamines make people feel good.

However, movement does not lie. One can move better or one cannot. Movement with **ease and confidence** is the SIGN of optimum central nervous system function. This is what we seek.

One needs to take note of the person who "appears" that he is executing the movement screen well, but in reality is making a really good replica. When I do movement screening I also check to see if

37

the person is BREATHING. Many a person will do the screen, but they accomplish the movement via breath-holding.

What we have observed sometimes is a person that stops breathing while performing basic movements; such as, getting up from a chair. Throughout the day, the person holds her breath to move. This to me is not a sign of good health, and could eventually lead into some possibly serious issues; such as heart disease.

The harder it is to perform life-skills, or execute the moves in the FMS, the more limited or handicapped the patient is. A person may have little or no pain, but if he cannot move, the body is telling me that he is in trouble, and is moving closer to illness and the eventual need for assistance. This bad trend could possibly lead to a hospital stay or having a nursing home as a permanent residence. Frequently, a nursing home resident has lost the basic skills required to take care of themself. The exam quickly highlights and identifies these losses so that we can intervene, retrain, strengthen, and restore ability.

A loss of mobility like grandma experienced DOES NOT happen overnight! It is slow and progressive. We don't "feel" ourselves gaining or losing weight. We don't feel a loss of motion. To the brain, MOTION or MOVEMENT is of the highest importance. Movement screening evaluates *movement*, most basic to our survival.

Evaluation and measurement of life-skills are great tools to use in explaining to patients the challenges and severity of their condition. Movement does not lie. A person moves well, or a person does not move well; "motion" or "movement" is life. I cannot think of a better barometer to evaluate health. We all innately understand when "mom" or "grand pop" is not moving well, that our loved one has an issue. Restore "movement" and, quite often, the other things resolve.

"Motion is Life... life is motion." ~ Dr. Dejarnette

CHAPTER FOUR

THE POWER WITHIN... BREATH

The body, as I have already stated, is a wonderful machine. When the body is healthy and trained to reach its full potential, the results can be fantastic. There are people and cultures throughout the world which confound our Western scientific explanations. Learning is great, but at times can be limiting. Here in Western civilization, we test and prove everything. Yet, some things man does cannot be quantified with our current technology. In a *Discovery Channel* presentation called, *"Mysteries of the Mind"* Tibetan Monks were shown making steam in subzero weather. These monks take a wet sheet, meditate in sub-zero temperatures, and make steam.

This phenomenon defies Western thinking. We cannot prove how it happens, but it happens. Most people in the West would be suffering from hypothermia under such circumstances. However, these monks have trained themselves to overcome the elements by tapping into some of the body's unique power systems.

Another example of this superhuman power is demonstrated by the Shaolin Monks who resist spears with their necks and break bricks with their hands. They have trained their bodies to become human weapons, and have made their bones impervious to fracture after striking stone.

I wondered how they do such remarkable things. The answer is they train the body to perform to that potential, and tap the body's enormous resources of power. The body is an incredible machine that is not as fragile and disease prone as we have been taught. The body contains unbelievable power systems that warrant further study.

Most of us are somewhat familiar with the structure of the brain, and the heart. Western science is famous for stating we utilize just 10 percent of our brain's potential. That means 90% of the brain's potential is *untapped*. In the West, we also know about cardiovascular function, but fail to reach this system's potential. In the East, many healthcare practices and rituals focus on breathing. The West has overlooked, and failed to completely understand and develop this unique system of power and potential.

I remember observing paper-thin diaphragms in the cadavers we studied in gross dissection lab. In the East, diaphragms in cadavers have been measured to be about a half inch thick according to Daniel Ried, author of *Chi Gung, Harnessing the Power of the Universe*. According to Eastern medical thought, the diaphragm acts as a second heart when used to its potential. The diaphragm aids in oxygenating the blood, and assists the heart in moving blood throughout the body. The development of the diaphragm muscle taps an energy system in the body that does many fantastic and wonderful things.

By utilizing a more developed diaphragm, the body rids itself of toxins faster, increases the amount of oxygen in the body, and activates the *parasympathetic* nervous system. In the book, *Stress Free for Good,* by Dr. Fred Luskin and Dr. Kenneth R. Pelletier; they note that "deep breathing" can be as effective as two blood pressure medications.

Short and shallow breathing are signs of "stress". Ever see a dog pant? The dog does not look relaxed does it? Panting or "short and shallow" breathing are signs the body is overloaded or "locked into" a part of the nervous system called the *sympathetic*.

The sympathetic nervous system is needed to rouse energy, but if it ramps up too high then the heart beats too fast and we can develop hypertension, strokes and heart attacks.

There is another nervous system called *parasympathetic* or the "rest and digest" part of the body. It is like the "yin" of the yin/yang. Yin is more feminine or "soft" and man is the "yang" or "hard" aspect of the yin/yang relationship. Each has its place, but an imbalance in the nervous system such as, being stuck in the sympathetic system, causes way too much adrenaline flow and other hormone imbalances. We don't want to be too far into yin or parasympathetics either, or else we will be lethargic and monotone.

Fitness and exercise helps develop the sympathetic nervous system, but we also need to learn to relax.

In today's culture, many of us have activated our sympathetic nervous systems without being engaged in physical activity. We know this system is the one utilized in *flight or fight* responses, which activates during athletic competition, exercise, and manual labor. Instead, we turn on the sympathetic nervous system as we sit at our desk, in our cars and at other inappropriate times. We have taught or conditioned the brain to utilize this system at the wrong time.

A simple observation of the most prescribed medications reveals that half of them are for anxiety and depression. It is estimated that 70-80 percent of the adult population is currently taking some form of medication and most are for anxiety and/or depression. Some of the other top medications prescribed are for sleep disturbances, pain, digestive disorders, high blood pressure, and cardiac arrhythmias, etc. All of these medications are designed to address the **symptoms** of an out-of-control sympathetic nervous system, e.g. stress.

The medications use different metabolic pathways to control the out-of-control system but most people who have "high blood pressure" will continue to "manage" the condition the rest of their lives via medications. How the "out of control sympathetic overload" presents symptoms can vary from person to person. Then a person is "diagnosed" with a condition such as ulcerative colitis and then "treated" for the condition.

The power systems of sympathetics and parasympathetics, if imbalanced, create all kinds of dysfunctional hormone activity. Many things could lead to this phenomenon; I am not limiting this to structural alignment alone.

Worry, fears/phobias, conditioned responses via the subconscious, foods, too much TV, news, etc. could all be contributors; even excessive exercise or habitual area-specific exercise.

Area-specific meaning, Susie runs for exercise 5 miles per day, and that is all Susie does. I am not saying "running" is bad, but Susie could also incorporate some strength training, Yoga, rock climbing or some other exercise routine.

The CNS loves learning new things and variety. Being "habitual" is good to some degree but can also cause imbalances. Literally... the term "stuck in a rut" is what happens with overtraining or a lack of some diversity in a person's health strategy. The brain creates almost a groove or "rut" for the activity. Too much of something is

NOT good; be it running or eating broccoli. The "too much" effect creates stress, and could lead to anxiety.

With the amount of medication Americans consume and the "high rates" of anxiety and depression, alarm bells should be going off in our heads at those staggering figures. Life is supposed to be a gift. Somehow, life has turned into a rat-race of survival that ends in the hospital or nursing home. Our stomachs are upset and our minds are upset due to an imbalance in the nervous system known as stress (sympathetic overload).

Neurologically we only have two primal fears: the fear of falling and the fear of loud noises. That means all of our other phobias and anxieties are learned. We have trained ourselves to be scared. We have not utilized the great powers within us; instead, we have trained them to work against us.

"Fear is an illusion." ~ Michael Jordan

If we start tapping our energy systems and allocate them appropriately, we can enjoy miraculous healings, incredible athletic feats, and have a far greater appreciation and enjoyment of life itself.

To make full use of the *Miracles in Minutes* techniques we need an understanding of the resources of power and healing generated by our own energy systems. One of those untapped energy systems is breathing. I have briefly talked about breathing and in particular *diaphragmatic* breathing. Many pain syndromes like low back pain, neck pain, and headaches have to do with faulty breathing patterns. Some doctors and healers believe that all illness is due to faulty breathing or a lack of oxygen.

Headaches, in particular, for many are due to a lack of oxygen to the brain. Short, shallow breathing triggers the sympathetic nervous system, which activates muscle tissue for work. Instead, we sit and stress-out. This phenomenon creates a cycle of pain by releasing more stress hormones, which increases our stressed-out thinking, leading to a plethora of maladies. By simply engaging diaphragmatic breathing, we can relieve headaches, low back pain, and most neck pain in minutes. Notice I did not say "cure," but "relieve." I think we would all agree breathing is essential to life. So, wouldn't improper or faulty breathing negatively impact health?

If you are a doctor, therapist, personal trainer or health instructor then ask your patient/client to take a deep breath and notice what moves. If you are a patient and are using this book at home then stand in front of the mirror and take a deep breath.

I'll bet the neck moves, and not the belly. When people chest-breathe, they tend to activate the scalene (neck) muscles to lift and move the chest. These little muscles are secondary movers and breathing assistants, not primary breathing muscles. Hence, the wrong muscle is doing the job. The pain produced is a signal that this is occurring. In this instance, it is not a neck problem or head-ache that needs treatment, but a faulty breathing pattern that needs to be corrected.

This is where I have deviated from typical care paths. I am NOT treating the symptoms such as neck pain or headaches. Simplified, the body's basic needs are:

1. **Air**
2. **Food**
3. **Water**
4. **Shelter**

And the hierarchy is simple… air/breathing is first; for without it we would only be here about 5 minutes max. Food, water, and shelter can be related to movement. We need to move to obtain these things essential for life. So basically we have AIR and MOVEMENT, which is dependent on structural alignment and functions of the brain/body connection.

Faulty breathing, or stressed breathing might be a learned habit. So to restore health or eliminate pain, we need to evaluate authentic breathing; Is a person still breathing when one moves? So I evaluate breathing while sitting and standing, and again during the FMS. Breathing is *NUMERO UNO* to life. Breathing is our FIRST exercise and last... we inhale our first breath, and exhale our last breath. No breath = no life. The question is: Is the person breathing deep and relaxed, or exhibiting a "stressed" or dysfunctional breathing method?

By learning the mechanics of *diaphragmatic breathing*, and then teaching the patient how to breathe properly, we can correct many of our patients' conditions. This type of breathing calms the mind, relaxes the muscles, and brings a sense of ease to mind, body, and spirit. Of course, as doctors, we learn much about the physical component, very little about the mental, and none about the spiritual. The spiritual is left up to the shaman, rabbi, priest, or minister. It is my opinion that we need healing of the whole man: body, mind, and spirit.

Breathing is also part of meditation in many religions. Some may have issue with relaxing or deep breathing or the term, "meditation". But if one does, then let's consider that prayer is like a conversation... one speaks, and the other listens. If we are always speaking (active mind), then when does the person "hear" or listen to WISDOM?

The atheist or *pure scientist* could recognize the fact that the prefrontal cortex is most active when we are relaxed. Either way.... being relaxed and diaphragmatic breathing is essential to health, and the prefrontal cortex is the smartest part of our brains. Despite having "great intelligence" a stressed-out person is not gaining full access to the prefrontal cortex.

PET scans show that depressed people have almost no activity in the prefrontal cortex. Happy people, or well-adjusted people, have very bright scans or activity levels in the prefrontal cortex. Deep breathing or diaphragmatic breathing allows the prefrontal cortex to "boot" back up or "turn on." No need to *freak out*... just breathe, and the answers will come.

Why is it that the underlying message of the Bible is... "Fear not, for I am with you." The SUPER INTELLIGENCE is the prefrontal cortex, and it is with us when we are at peace; breathing deeply and relaxed, and trusting in something greater than us.

This is just something to consider for reasons to why we evaluate breathing, and WHY we practice this discipline in the healthcare arena or for success and happiness in life. Breath is the KEY to accessing super mental intelligence, health, healing, and emotional intelligence. Breath helps us rule over our emotions, rather than allowing our emotions ruling over us.

Diaphragmatic breathing allows a normal reset to the nervous system, thus allowing a return to nervous system balance and hormonal balance.

The Chinese take breathing a step further with **Chi Gung** (also spelled Qi-qong and Chi Kung). The Chinese practice this type of breathing for healing and a peaceful mind.

In India, the great Yogis also spend a lot of their discipline on breathing. The Yogis refer to this as Prana, while the Chinese call it Chi. We get our word for breathing (from spirit) by the word respiration, or *re-spirit-intaking*. Spirit, in theological terms, states the spirit brings life. I think we can all agree that if we stop breathing, or re-spirit-intaking long enough, we will not be living.

Generally, people understand that proper breathing during exercise is important. People are also familiar with Yoga, which also emphasizes breathing in its discipline. The foundation of most traditional Chinese medicine started with exploring proper breathing, and different breathing techniques.

The Chi Gung method incorporates the "inner core". Many people today are familiar with *core training* but few realize the body has TWO CORES. The inner-core is made up of AUTONOMIC or "automatic" neurological sequencing patterns that are beyond conscious involvement.

Conscious involvement means thinking. Our heart beats via the unconscious mind. We do not have to "think" or consciously make our heart beat. Movement also should occur naturally and not consciously. A small child does NOT think about walking to get a cookie. The child just walks. Movement in a human is painful when the inner core is not sequencing properly due to an issue.

The inner core is made up of the diaphragm, transversus abdominous (think of a corset or back brace), *multifidi* (small little muscles attached to the spine) and the pelvic floor. As people get older, in America, many develop issues with the pelvic floor, with signs or symptoms of:

- **Incontinence (need of an adult diaper)**
- **Sexual dysfunction**
- **Impotence**
- **Low back pain**

The Chinese breathing method incorporates the inner core into their practice. Upon inhalation, they take the breath in and then

49

close the anal sphincter, tighten the lower abs, and close the epi-glottis (throat). After that, they hold the breath, pack Chi energy (spirit or breath) into organs, and then move it around with the mind. **This breathing method is only for the advanced student and practitioner to use.** The method is called *Iron Shirt Chi Kung*. I am not going any further into this subject because of problems that could arise from this type of breathing. I am merely making one aware of some unique practices.

The breathing utilized here is diaphragmatic breathing. I recom-mend you start with the patient in the supine position, if possible and have him take a deep abdominal breath and breathing into the floor or back. The stomach should rise and inflate into the low back. It is as if the patient is blowing up a balloon in his abdomen. The patient can place his hand about one and a half inches below the umbilicus (belly button) and imagine breathing into his hand. Upon exhalation, the umbilicus should fall toward the spine.

It is important that the patient inhale slowly and gently. **One can start with a 4 second inhale relaxed and deeply followed by a 6 second exhale, followed by 2 seconds of non-breathing. Repeat this method for 2 minutes** and then slowly over time increase the times but keep exhalation longer than inhalation. Most people are OVER BREATHING, or breathing too much.

A deep breath is not a forced breath, but a gentle asking of air to flow into the body. Think of the type of breathing right before falling to sleep. It is a slow, smooth, and even flow of air into the lungs over about three to five seconds; followed by a gentle, slow, and smooth release last-ing five to seven seconds. As the patient improves his breathing tech-nique and strengthens the diaphragm, inhalations and exhalations can increase to a ten-to-fifteen-second duration. It is important to breathe slowly, smoothly, deeply, and steadily. As the patient progresses, he can use this technique in a sitting and standing position.

50

Forced breathing turns the sympathetic nervous system on again or increases the degree that it is on. You see power-breathing used by power lifters, boxers, and football players. Rapid, powerful breathing is for combat, not healing.

When diaphragmatic breathing is done properly, the body will absorb more oxygen and expel more toxins while triggering alpha waves in the brain. Alpha waves stimulate creativity and relaxation. This one simple exercise can reduce stress, help us lose weight, improve organ health, and alleviate pain.

If you have never experienced diaphragmatic breathing, you will discover how liberating it can be but also how challenging it can be. You will learn that—just like your patients—you have been breathing improperly. Daily practice of this method will give the patient and you what most people desire . . . peace-of-mind and body relaxation. It is like a self-applied massage of mind, body, and spirit when done correctly. Upon mastery of this skill, the patient may feel warmth at the spot located below the belly button. Now the patient is moving energy in the body effectively.

If we really studied breathing, or *re-spirit-intaking*, we would notice some very interesting and fascinating things. Our bodies are like a baffle, or an accordion, bringing in air, (expanding), and then letting out air, (contracting).

With that observation, we will note that the body moves rhythmically forward and back, and I believe in a very particular rhythm. The movement is precise and stored in the brain's data bank of normal parasympathetic breathing. This is my theory, but I believe the brain has a storage bank of data containing normal/healthy frequency waves for body-tissues and organs.

The normal frequencies would be somewhat dependent on structural alignment. Optimal alignment can allow optimal function.

A car that is "tuned up" runs more efficient than a car that is out of *alignment*, and the mechanical timing of the engine is off from factory specifications. Any disruption of the body's normal alignment will make breathing more labored, and the body will respond in kind, with symptoms. Likewise, faulty breathing would affect alignment.

The reason this occurs is because breathing or respiration also plays a vital role in moving Cerebral Spinal Fluid (CSF) through the central nervous system by a coordination of breathing and cranial sacral motion (skull/tailbone). CSF is the fluid that is examined during a "spinal tap" for meningitis. The Chinese have known about the CSF system for thousands of years.

CSF is the nuclear fuel of the brain's nuclear reactor. CSF contains twice as much glycogen as our blood. The body runs on glucose, and an infant's brain utilizes 75 percent of all the glucose in the body. CSF fluid is specific to the brain and central nervous system. We might be able to conclude that the brain utilizes CSF for its power source.

The cranial sacral pump might be the *fountain of youth* that man has been looking for. It flows in the *river* of our spine and *fountains* in the brain. This source of power is stored in the abdomen.

Like any fountain, it has a pool at the bottom that needs a pump to push the fluid to the top. Life started with an abdominal attachment known as the umbilical cord. The abdomen is where life grows, namely, babies. Abdominal movement and hip movement are where all athletic power comes from. Hip transfer or hip movement is what enables us to hit a homerun, a golf ball, knock someone's lights out, or procreate. When CSF flow and breathing synchronize, perfect balance in the body is facilitated. This synchronization creates miraculous healing and a feeling of wellness. The feeling can only be described with a theological term: Heaven.

When all of the body's power systems are lined up and in harmony, the body will feel almost ethereal, weightless, light, and joyous. It is as if the body is *smiling* on the inside, which is difficult to contain and explain. To reach this nirvana, the body has to be in proper structural alignment, balanced between sympathetic and parasympathetic nervous systems, and consuming a healthy diet.

The body is in constant need of energy and that energy needs to flow with as little resistance as possible. We need to exercise, eat right, breathe correctly, and be in alignment, to experience Optimum Health.

The exercises that enable the body to work in concert, are called functional exercises. There are certain muscles that should work together to perform certain actions. This is how most movement occurs. However, when muscles become weak, or we execute movements with bad form, the body remembers that and then begins to utilize a faulty movement pattern. For example, picture someone walking with one foot turned out to the side. That is a faulty movement pattern.

Functional training re-patterns the body to operate according to its proper specifications, such as when the foot points straight ahead with the knee falling directly over the ankle. One cannot expect the body to operate properly if faulty movement patterns are not corrected. After a period of time, the brain adjusts to assume that walking with the foot turned out is the way the body should move. This is what it has been taught. By specifically retraining the body, and reminding the joint of all of its functions, the body will execute proper movement.

Pain is the voice the compensatory muscles use to say, "I have lost function, and I am not operating properly. I am wearing unevenly because the load is not being evenly distributed. Help me!"

The purpose of this book is to give the doctor, therapist, or patient a simple and safe method of eradicating pain and returning function in the least amount of time. The topics covered in this chapter merit books unto themselves to fully appreciate the complexities and nuances of their use. If you agree that **breathing, exercise, alignment, function, and stretching** are valid methods to employ to improve body function, then you will make good use of the information provided.

The beauty of utilizing these methods lies in the fact that there is not a right or wrong sequence to apply these methods and achieve results. You could start with breathing to produce the outcome, or you could start with stretches and still get great results; or better yet, you could combine the two. You could start in the ankle and work your way up, or you could start in the core and work your way out. Both methods work. The patient will provide the starting point in which a stimulus is removed or introduced into one of the energy systems of the body. By allowing the energy to flow freely in the body, we allow the power within to do its job. That job is to heal, repair, rejuvenate, and establish *nirvana* in the "temple of man."

CHAPTER FIVE

THE WAY-OF-LIFE FORCE

When we talk about life what are we really talking about? I think the best, one-word answer is *energy*. Energy can be described as constant motion. We can see the properties of energy demonstrated in the wind and ocean waves. When energy is restricted or disrupted it dies, moves away, or builds up and explodes.

The way-of-life force is my observation of nature and how life energy works. Life-force seems to follow a pattern. Somehow, two elements unite to become one. The new, united element, starts out small, and rapidly becomes larger; thereby, creating more systems and tools for a specific purpose.

This life-force phenomenon typically follows what I call, *The Flower Principle*. A seed meets earth, water, and light and begins its journey toward becoming a flower. The seed opens and establishes a root network to sustain and extrapolate energy sources for its life expression.

After establishing its root network, it breaks through the soil and grows straight toward the sun. It continues developing its root network to secure its place among the living and gathers more resources to enable it to blossom. The plant soon develops buds as it stores and retrieves energy from its root structure while being nourished by the atmosphere and sunlight. The plant takes in carbon dioxide, expels oxygen, and turns sunlight into photogenic energy, which we call *photosynthesis*. The root system feeds the plant nutrients and water from the soil.

The plant has now gathered all the resources necessary to bloom. Its bud opens, revealing to the world its inner beauty and the potential it harbored from the time it was a seed. Once it has reached its potential, it slowly withers, wilts, and fades into the ground from which it came.

The human life force follows much the same pattern. We stand upright, and our shoulders are back, our legs are straight, and we are in perfect alignment. Now as a man's strength withers, his knees pin together while getting out of a chair. His pelvis is rotated anterior and the mid-back increases its kyphosis, or hunchback, as the head pushes forward. The weight of the head will eventually increase the thoracic curve and the man will quickly move closer to his ultimate sentence . . . death. Man appears to be moving back into the seed format.

How—and why—does this occur? My theory is that we sit too much. We may have evolved intellectually, but no one told our bodies. Our bodies are designed as a hunter-gatherer and survival-man machine. We were designed to climb, jump, run, lift, and move in all kinds of wonderful ways. Instead, we sit. We sit in school, at work, at home, and in the car, on our way to work; which has created muscular atrophy, tight hips, and abnormal movement patterns.

The application of pressure over time is the principle an orthodontist uses to correct the spacing and alignment of teeth. I believe that the pressure of sitting exerted over a long period of time, combined with underdevelopment of the glute muscles, has caused the femurs, or thigh bones, to move to the front of the hip joint. This has created a misaligned hip joint, decreased the range of motion of the hip, and caused the beginning of improper biomechanical function. How many people get hip replacements in this country?

It is also highly likely that the first shoes we wore inhibited motion. Most baby shoes laced above our ankles and the soles were extremely hard, which prevented the development of the stabilizing muscles of the ankle. The muscles of the feet never developed to their potential. A good example of feet muscles that are developed to their potential can be found by observing a female gymnast. A gymnast on the balance beam is something amazing to watch because their feet grip the balance beam like a hand grips a ball. Can your feet do that?

Our pattern for walking is off from the beginning and perhaps this explains why we have so many surgeries for hip and knee replacements, foot problems, low-back pain, and somatic aches and pains. We got off on the *wrong foot* from the start, literally, and trained ourselves to use faulty movement patterns.

Those movement patterns stay with us throughout life because we do not know to correct them. A simple observation of the elderly explains this principle. First, observe the tone of their glutes or "buttocks". Notice their glute muscles are not developed. In other words, they have no backside whatsoever. They are hunched over, their head is front of their body, their knees pin together when they get out of a chair, their feet are spread apart, and when they walk... they take very tiny steps. They cannot move, are totally out of normal human alignment, and have lost the ability to balance.

The head is so far in front of the body that the falling signal from the cochlea (ear) makes it hard to balance. This further explains the mental confusion, forgetfulness, shaking hands and wide stance. Can you really expect them to relate to us if the brain is so concerned with deciphering whether they are falling? Do you think this mal-position might be affecting the CSF flow to the brain? If the brain is not getting adequate CSF flow, what do you think happens?; dizziness, fatigue, and memory problems. Is it starting to make sense?

After observing an elderly person's posture, it is simple to explain their other maladies. Since man's body is designed to walk upright, shortness of breath, dizziness, confusion, fatigue, headaches, knee pain, heart problems, bladder problems, etc. are logical complaints that result from the body trying to function from its bent position. Not one thing in this system is functioning the way it is designed to function. What's worse, we ignored the initial warning signs of malfunction. We just kept using bad form and bad technique, thinking it would have no impact on the body's ability to function in our later years. There's no need to wonder why we look and feel the way we do in our old age.

It is not very uplifting, but these observations provide some great insight into the cycle of life and the cycle of death, and an explanation of what happens to our bodies as we age.

The philosophy behind the *Miracles in Minutes* method is to bring man into his *flowering* position and sustain it for as long as possible by keeping the body in its proper alignment followed by re-patterning natural motion and movements. By simply implementing the rules of life, it is possible to extend life, while removing or diminishing the infirmities that plague us.

C H A P T E R   S I X

DIAGNOSTIC THERAPEUTIC TREATMENT

After completing the exam, I move into what I call: *diagnostic therapeutic treatment*. I evaluate the patient's use of foundational core muscles and note whether there is **symmetry, ease of motion, or tightness**. I also pay close attention to whether muscular tightness produces pain and whether stretching the muscle produces relief. **Any movement or stretch that produces relief is repeated.** I am a big believer in Pareto's Law, or the "80/20" principle. A little 20% stretch and/or exercise that produces 80% relief. Most care paths are the inverse… 80% effort with only 20% relief.

Treatment is geared towards the symptom:

Patient: "I have neck pain."

Doctor/therapist: "Oh, you MUST have a neck problem."

That is a myopic approach. If neck pain, then neck problem. I used to use this same philosophy but what I found was this… it takes FOREVER to get relief. The relief is usually very minor… 10-20%, and takes lots of time. That violates Pareto's law, or the 80/20 principle.

The typical approach for a neck problem is a heating pad to the neck, massages, rubs, creams and all kinds of care for the "neck problem". I did that for years but was unsatisfied with the results. It was not until I attended a continuing education seminar and the presenting doctor said something that STUCK with me... *"Typically, what is CAUSING the problem or symptom is FAR away from the area of pain."*

So the "diagnostic therapeutic treatment" means I am looking for the stretch or exercise that PRODUCES the greatest results with the least effort. The RESULT determines the care... *"Hey, that worked great and it only took 20 seconds!"* I use the result to determine the diagnosis. What helped alleviate the pain is what the care path is, or the treatment.

Any movement or stretch that causes pain or produces symptoms is discontinued immediately! The painful thing may give us a diagnosis; e.g., a "herniated disc", but the issue I had with that approach is this... not every person with a herniated L5 disc responds to the L5 herniated disc exercise or care suggestion. How many people have low-back surgery for the "herniated disc" and still have pain?

The answer is LOTS! It is so common that there is a new diagnosis and it is called "failed low-back surgery," for someone who STILL has low back pain despite surgery. I am not saying that ALL surgeries are bad or that surgery does not help. I am making the point that sometimes surgery does not work even though the herniation is visible on MRI.

The same can be said for stretches, exercises, physical therapy and chiropractic. Just because a stretch for low-back pain worked on our friend "Jane", who also has a herniated disc, does not mean that it will work for "Sally". If low-back pain care was that simple then low-back pain would be eradicated by now, but it is not.

It is not that a particular stretch is bad, but rather that it may be bad at that time, or is not what is needed. I believe the issue is that as humans we start with an amorphous goal to merely "do something" such as exercise because... *exercise is good for us.*

So when we have a "pain" we take an action step and "do something" which could be call a doctor, exercise, or some other "activity". The intention is very good but we need to measure the success of the "action step" to determine if the step is producing the result.

The *Miracles in Minutes* method seeks to measure the outcomes or outputs of activity. We cannot assume anything when someone is in pain or apply blanket-methods of care prescriptions. We specifically measure or quantify the "pain" and a person's ability to move with ease. Any activity, stretch or exercise that requires little effort and produces maximum results is the exercise or stretch of choice.

Diagnostic therapeutic treatment means the TREATMENT; whatever it is—including the weird, esoteric, left-ankle stretch to help the right shoulder pain or whatever—is on the table. **The "thing to do" is the thing that works!**

The trouble we get into as patients and doctors is "assuming". We think we know. Be open to everything.

Patient: "I have a herniated disc in my back and 10 years of low-back pain."

Doctor: "What have you done for it?"

Patient: "Medications to function, physical therapy, surgery, chiropractic, braces, massage, etc."

Doctor: "10 years of back therapy and no relief?"

Patient: "Yes... do you think you can help?"

Doctor: "Hmm... is it possible you don't have a back problem?"

61

Patient: "No... it hurts and it is definitely a back pain problem."

Doctor: "But ALL the care has been directed to the BACK and I am wondering... if maybe something ELSE is causing your back to hurt? Maybe, an old ankle problem?"

Patient: "That is insane! It is my back that hurts."

Doctor: "This is true, your back hurts, but it looks like this is a total violation of Pareto's law... 99% effort and cost and very little result... the back pain remains. "Insanity is doing the SAME THINGS and EXPECTING a different result."

ASSUME NOTHING, BUT BE OPEN
TO ANYTHING... that works!

Just because something hurts does not mean it is the issue or "problem." If the issue has not resolved then we need to explore other options and other areas. Part of my diagnostic therapeutic treatment is a quick "check" of common issues that can enable rapid results for many people. As noted, one does NOT have to do everything or anything that I am suggesting. These are merely SUGGESTIONS and apply the 80/20 principle, or little effort and maximum result, as the goal.

Let's Begin...

Look... listen... the MEB 3 is looking at big muscles, and the primary joints, such as the hips, and is assessing whether the left hip moves like the right and vice versa. Does doing this stretch as the *Miracles in Minutes* philosophical treatise help or not?

Care is not a "right" or "wrong" method. As I have been stressing all along: It is what stretch, exercise, breathing method or strength training method PRODUCE... the 80% relief with the 20% effort. In short, it is working "smart" vs. working hard.

If the left shoulder is stretched and a person with low back pain goes from a 10/10 to a 1/10 on the VAS, then who cares? It worked... it produced the result and the body can connect various muscles-to-muscles via a neural network to do almost anything.

Diagnostic therapeutic treatment is to get the doctor, the therapist and patient to THINK OUTSIDE THE BOX. Observe, measure (does it work or help, and if so, how much? 80%... bingo!)

The stretching pattern I use is something I call MEB 3, which refers to muscle (m), energy (e) and balance (b). MEB 3 focuses on releasing the most common malfunctioning compensatory core muscles to allow the body to move freely again. It is like an accelerated yoga class. We produce effects similar to those achieved during an hour's worth of yoga in about 15 minutes, by targeting the most common malfunctioning muscles with a specific stretching technique.

Let me explain how I use this process to identify a patient's problem: The first stretch I have the patient do is for the glutes. This stretch also reveals hip integrity or how "healthy" the hip is.

The hips are our "center of gravity" for the body. Where the hips go... the body goes. At least, that is what my football coach told me.

If the patient cannot internally rotate the leg at all, you will also find a positive Thomas' test and Patrick's test. For the layperson, these tests, Thomas and Patrick, help a doctor determine whether a patient has arthritis of the hip, tight muscles, or other problems. The "health" of the hip can determine a lot about the overall health of a person.

The hips are what LIFT US UP, center us and create tremendous lifting power and strength. Pinching, tightness, clicking, cramping and poor-moving hips wreak havoc on the body... everywhere. The hip does not complain much until it is too late. But the MEB 3 stretching and assessment can help a person or doctor quickly determine how well someone is.

The poorer the hip movement, or "clicking" and "tightness" in the hip joint, the more health issues someone typically has. The glute stretch helps to see what the hip is doing from one angle and may warrant some more evaluation and care paths. Think of the "glute stretch" as evaluating the hip socket.

The next stretch/assessment is for the psoas. The psoas, a muscle located in the abdomen that connects to the hip, often times becomes very tight and also very weak. Tight psoas, also known as a "hip flexor", can cause lots of problems throughout the body.

Hip flexion means to bring the knee towards the chest. Pinching in the front of the hip is NOT a good thing. The hip is "impinged" or the capsule that lubricates the hip is inflamed. The psoas stretch or test is looking at the health of the front of the hip as well as a possible SOLUTION to alleviate pain.

If someone has a severely deteriorated hip do NOT stretch the psoas. Severe hip arthritis needs to be seen by a specialist such as an Orthopedist. If someone is doing the psoas stretch and tears are coming to one's eyes... the hip is probably shot.

Start slowly, or do a "little" and check the result in using the stretches and exercises I am about to "suggest". If we JUMP IN full steam and do not measure and assume that "this stretch" will work for "x" condition, then we are not being safe. Do a little bit and if the pain number is going up, such as a 6/10 is now a 7/10, then stop. However if the pain number is going down then we can do a little more, and see if that the person is moving in the right direction.

The MEB system uses PNF, or a "contract and relax," type of stretching. The person is taken to the stretch position and then "contracts" the muscle against resistance for a period of time. Then the person relaxes, for say, 20 seconds as they are stretched to a new range. The cycle repeats stretching against resistance for about 30 seconds, followed by relaxing and stretching.

The goal of the contraction phase is not for the patient to contract maximally, but at about **20-50%** of the muscles' potential. This is the PNF method I primarily use, but there are at least two others. You may research them online or find them in other books. They work well, but I find this style to be the most efficient, and it is part of the system I have developed.

The MEB3 method uses the PNF (contract and relax) method of stretching and is a quick way to alleviate many pains. We achieve this just by placing someone into these big stretching patterns.

If you are a layperson and reading this and are confused, then simply go to the CONDITION sections such as "neck pain" or "low-back pain." An advanced personal-trainer and professional will understand this section for rehabilitation. If one so chooses to utilize this method then please proceed slowly. Remember: Follow the commandments!

For the professional, no matter what the patient's complaint, I try to get him to apply this MEB 3 method first; unless the patient cannot tolerate it. In my experience, very few patients have been unable to tolerate this diagnostic therapeutic method. The severe acute patient is where skill and experience come into play. If a person has a hard time sitting, then try wall sits first.

Wall sits... the old gym class favorite. Place one's back against a wall. Walk the feet out so that when the person "sits" or "squats" the knees are at 90 degrees. Who would have thought that if a person cannot sit in a chair or on an exam table that having them perform a wall sit would alleviate the pain for most people in less than 2 minutes? It works for most, but not "all" people.

Do what works—nothing more and nothing less. This is "diagnostic therapeutic treatment."

CHAPTER SEVEN

MEB 3 Exercises

Ever since I was a child, I loved finding patterns. I loved games like *find the word* and would do them incessantly. This love of patterns, and figuring out the riddle, helped me find what I call MEB 3.

I began to notice that most patients had certain muscles that were tight and when I stretched them, the patient improved. I kept learning new things and new stretches, and one day I thought I found a pattern that made me feel great; and many pains I was feeling went away almost instantly. The feeling I experienced after it was done was hard to explain. I just knew I felt awesome. I felt light, tall, agile, mobile and younger.

I soon began to apply these specific stretches on my patients. They too, began to experience what I felt. Many patients did not have words to explain their feelings, but many felt improvement, and the pain they had disappeared almost instantly.

At that point I knew I was on to something. I started seeing high degrees of predictability in problems and conditions, but also some unexpected results in some patients with certain problems. It was the unexpected; sometimes bad, results that lead me to establish the rules, or what I call: *Dr. Wood's commandments*. The commandments enable anyone to use the MEB 3 protocol with positive results.

I established the order of the stretches because it allows the doctor and patient to use less time to do more. The patient has to make few position changes and sets up a quick exam for the doctor at the same time. The doctor can use the stretches to determine what is wrong rather quickly, and have an idea how to correct the issue of pain; almost instantly. Here is what I have found to work effectively and efficiently:

Number 1: Glutes. The glute stretch starts with the patient in a supine position. The leg is then brought across the body at about a 45-degree angle and pressed toward the floor. The stretch can be adjusted to increase the leg angle by pointing the knee towards the shoulder or decrease the leg angle, (knee more toward foot), for the extremely tight, or those in extreme pain.

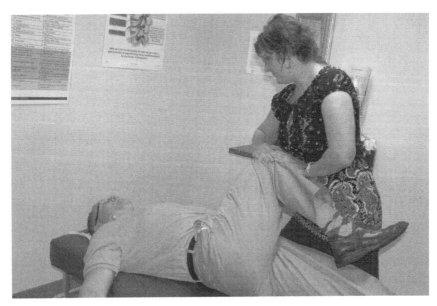

(Glute/buttock stretch, or back of the hip socket stretch)

This stretch should ONLY be felt in the glutes, or buttocks. If the patient complains of low back pain or groin pain (seen in women mainly) stop the stretch immediately. We are stretching the buttocks, not the back or groin. Pain is an indication that the body is blocking or cannot move properly to allow the stretch to be correctly performed. If the practitioner continues, the patient could be in worse shape than when he started. Why? Let's re-examine my commandments:

1. **Never create or reproduce the symptoms that brought the patient into the office!**
2. **Always respect the Great Physician/Innate Intelligence (yes is *yes*, and no is *no*)!**
3. **Always use perfect form and technique.**

Now for some reason women will have groin restriction, blocking the stretch. Many women feel tightness in the front of their hip when taking the leg across the body. If you PNF the psoas, most of the time we can resume the glute stretch with the stretching sensation occurring in the buttocks. This stretch is a great way to relieve low-back and Sacroiliac (SI) pain. For the layman/patient, the SI is one of the main load-bearing joints in the body, and makes up part of its (body) foundation. To find the SI joint, simply place your hands on your hips/pelvis. Now reach your thumbs back in an attempt to touch each other. The things sticking out or bumps you feel are the Sacroiliac joints.

Number 2: Piriformis/hip capsule. The second stretch I do is for the hip capsule and piriformis. The piriformis is the muscle that turns the foot outward (or external rotation) and is one of the main compensatory muscles of the body. It is also a muscle that produces hip problems, foot problems, sciatica, and low-back pain. Non-moving, or *frozen*, hips inhibits the patient's power and CSF flow.

69

After completing the glute stretch, I have the patient place the ankle across the opposite knee. The patient is still supine (on one's back) and I have the patient push the knee toward the table using his leg muscles. A lot of patients try to use their hands to do this; but I want them to use their leg muscles since the leg muscles move the leg and not the arm muscles. The patient should hold the stretch anywhere from 30 seconds–2 minutes.

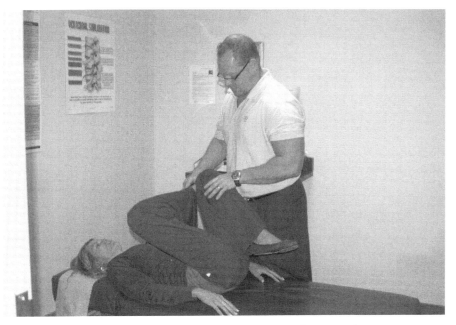

(Piriformis or posterior hip capsule stretch)

Then I have the patient relax, and I approximate the leg towards the head in that exact same position. This stretches the piriformis and the hip capsule. The first movement was mainly for the hip capsule and some small functional retraining of the hip joint. The approximation of the hip is lengthening the piriformis.

Approximate the hip: means to bring knee closer to the chest while in this "figure 4" type position.

Hold the stretch anywhere from 30 seconds–2 minutes. The tighter the joint, the slower and longer the stretch. Do not forget the commandments! If the patient complains of back pain, stop immediately. We are stretching the hip, not the back. Spasms, pain, sciatica, or any pain even in the mid-back or neck are all signs to stop immediately.

Perform the glute and hip capsule/piriformis stretches on both sides of the body before moving to the third stretch. This is done for efficiency of time and a good comparison. How is the person's hip is moving? Which side is tighter? On which side is the patient complaining of pain? Make notes and attempt to even the hips out. Do not expect this to occur in one visit. Just hold the tight side for a longer period of time to start creating balance in the body.

Number 3: Hip/low-back release/lateral line release. The third stretch is for the erector spinae, tensor fascia late, and iliotibial band. Pay special attention to detail when implementing this stretch because it can be a miracle, or a nightmare. This stretch is also contraindicated for people with hip replacements. You can modify it by grabbing the pelvis instead of using the leg as a fulcrum. The pelvis, and not hip or leg; if you do not know the difference between the two, then do not do it at all.

Have the patient lie on her side. The body should be at a 45-degree angle. The bottom arm needs to be behind the patient as if she is swimming. The patient's other hand should grasp the bottom part of the exam table or bench. Place your hand directly above the knee and hold the leg down and back toward the floor at a 45-degree angle. Then the patient pulls her body toward the floor/table at a 45-degree angle while you hold the leg secure. A stretching sensation will occur right above the SI joint into the latisumus dorsi and erector spinae and something Tom Meyers—a massage therapist who studied under Ida Rolfe—calls the lateral line.

If you are a layperson/patient let me define a couple of terms:

1. *SI or Sacroiliac:* This is one of the main joints that allow us to stand upright and walk. To find the joint place your hands on your hips. Now take your thumbs and have them reach for each other behind you. If you feel a bump then you have probably found the SI joint.

2. *Latismus dorsi:* This is a muscle that attaches to your arm and runs all the way to your pelvis. If you have ever seen a body builder put his hands on his hips and elbows out to the side to show how wide his back or "wings" are then you have seen the lats or latismus dorsi. Or maybe if you have ever seen the guys whose arms cannot rest against the sides of their body because their muscles stick out so much then you have seen the lats.

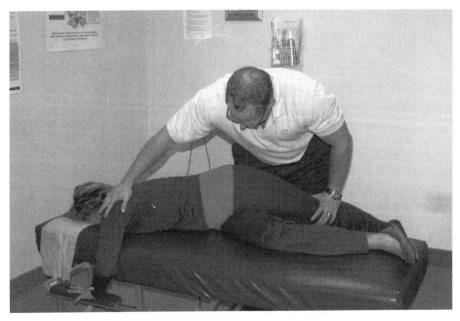

(Lateral line or erector spinae stretch)

You are on-target if the patient describes the sensation as feeling good, or if it is described as a *good pain*, or it brings about a sense of relief. If this is the case, continue the stretch for about 30 seconds. The patient will experience great results. During the relaxation phase, press the leg closer toward the ground at a 45-degree angle, while your other hand secures the rib cage or shoulder. Repeat two more times. If the patient complains of SI pain or back pain, then stop immediately and try repositioning the patient. These complaints might cease by rolling the patient more onto the front of the hip.

If pain persists after repositioning the patient, then stop immediately and do not try to repeat the stretch. This stretch can achieve miraculous results, but it also has the potential to cause the most harm of all the things I present in this book. If this stretch is done properly, the patient will immediately feel taller when she stands up. The other thing you will notice is lumbar flexion is now greatly improved. The patient may even be able to touch her toes. Significant improvement will occur in most cases.

The acute patient warrants the use of extreme caution when attempting this stretch because of its potential to make the person feel worse. Perform a gentle test and apply light pressure on any new patient or acute patient. Address any discomfort or pain by repositioning the patient. Again, if repositioning the patient does not relieve the discomfort or pain, stop the stretch immediately. If all is well, then perform the stretch on both sides. If one side of the body "complains" even though repositioning has been done, then stop, even if you have done one side without the patient complaining. Strict adherence to my commandments is necessary to prevent irritating the issue. Commit them to memory:

1. **Never create or reproduce the symptoms that brought the patient into the office!**

2. **Always respect the Great Physician/Innate... yes is *yes* and no is *no*!**
3. **Always use perfect form and technique.**

Number 4: Hip flexor/psoas stretch. In my description of an aging man's mal-position of anterior femurs and anterior tilted pelvis, the hip flexors play the biggest role. The iliopsoas connects to the anterior aspect of the lumbar spine and to the anterior aspect of the femur. Can you see how this muscle and the entire hip flexor group would shorten from sitting? Can you see how this muscle group would pull the pelvis and sacrum into an anterior or flexion position? Can you see how this muscle with the rest of the hip flexor group would bring the femur to the front of the joint?

What happens when a muscle contracts? It shortens. Muscles flex joints and extend joints. Muscles move bones. What happens if too much movement occurs or a muscle imbalance develops? In short; pain. If the muscle keeps contracting it will dislocate the joint, so the body elicits a pain response in an attempt to prevent this from occurring. Pain is not a bad thing; we just need to understand why it occurs and how to alleviate it.

Have the person sit on the edge of a table. Now have the person lie back and bring the knees to the chest while the hands hold the knees. The person is in the fetal position with the arms holding the knees to the chest.

Next the person will let one leg go and have the leg drop towards the floor. The other leg is still secured to the chest with the other arm. The doctor or therapist will place his hand over the patient's hand that is holding the knee to the chest and the other hand is placed just above the knee. If this makes one uncomfortable then the patient can just hold the leg.

The arm above the knee on the "down leg" will apply some resistance as the person attempts to raise the leg. The patient should only contract the muscle with about 20-50% effort for about 30 seconds. As the patient relaxes, the doctor or therapist will "stretch" the leg to a new range of motion. At the new range of motion the patient will contract again for about 30 seconds with about 20-50% effort. The patient relaxes and a light stretch towards the floor occurs.

Stay within a person's comfort zone of where she is most relaxed. Instruct her to breath and relax. Do three cycles and remember the rules... no joint pain! No nerve pain or numbness! Muscle stretching is fine, but a sensation of "tearing" is not!

A common complaint of low-back pain in a patient who works out by doing a lot of leg lifts is not the result of lower-abs work. Rather, the lower abdominal muscles are so weak that they compensate by using the hip flexors, thereby creating lumbar disc problems or SI problems. Most SI pain or lumbar pain vanishes as soon as the hip flexors are released. Ask your patients who complain of low back pain if they are doing leg lifts when they work out. If they are, then most likely it is the leg lifts that caused the back pain. If that exercise is causing the pain, the patient will typically get low-back pain that day or the next day. Leg lifts are not a bad exercise, but improper leg lifts can cause the patient to have a lot of pain.

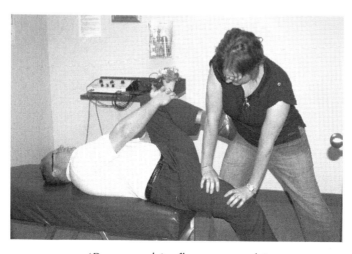

(Psoas or hip flexor stretch)

Number 5: Seated Pillow or Exercise Ball Squeeze. This exercise is a great way to relieve SI pain, neck pain, mid-back pain, low-back pain, and sciatica.

To perform this exercise, the patient should sit on a hard chair or table. Place a pillow folded in half, or an exercise ball, between the patient's knees. Make sure the patient's feet point straight ahead and rest on the floor and the legs are about shoulder width apart. The patient squeezes the pillow or exercise ball with her knees while the feet remain flat on the floor, repeating the motion 10 to 15 times. If there is no complaint of pain, the patient can repeat the motion until her legs feel as if they are working evenly on both sides. Stop the exercise immediately if the patient complains of pain.

If the exercise is done properly, the patient will feel straighter and taller. Additionally, the patient will be able to bend over and almost touch her toes.

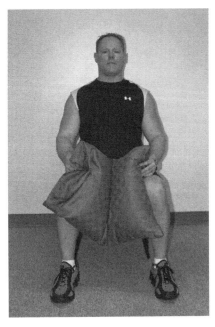

(Seated Pillow Squeezes)

Number 6: Wall sits or *Air chair.* This exercise is a great way to restore normal pelvic position. Surprisingly, this exercise also relieves arm pain, cervical radiculopathy (arm numbness or pain), low-back pain, mid-back pain and sciatica. How do we know if this is the right thing to do? By the way the patient's body responds to it. Does the patient have pain in this position, or is the pain decreasing? If there is no complaint of pain, then repeat the exercise.

Begin by asking the patient to place her back against a door, then have her walk her feet away from the door with the legs directly under the shoulders and hips. Next, the patient squats like she is going to sit on an invisible chair, slowly sinking down with the back flat against the door. If the patient cannot flatten her back against the door, just have her squat making sure the knees stay over the feet and ankles.

Many people tend to compensate by using the *adductor magnus*; the knees will move toward each other as if *knock-kneed.* This is incorrect. If the patient has complained of pain anywhere in her body, compare the initial complaint of pain to the level of pain while holding this position. For example, the patient has 9/10 "neck pain," and in the wall sit position the pain in the neck reduces to 4/10, then BINGO! We found it.

If the pain is reduced, then keep the patient in the position as long as humanly possible. This rule is the key to achieving miraculous results: *Any exercise or stretch that substantially relieves pain, reduces it quickly, improves function or range of motion; needs to be done until the pain resolves or reaches a tolerable threshold!*

The patient may complain that her leg muscles are fatigued. It is all right for a weak muscle(s) to complain if using it reduces the patient's debilitating pain. If the "exercise" alleviates a "body pain", explain that this is the position or movement that the body requires to heal itself.

If the patient's knees are hurting, then stop the exercise, or do not have the patient squat so far down. I typically have the patient start at a slight bend and move them down to almost parallel to the ground. If the knee pain is persistent, then stop this exercise.

Most importantly, check the patient's form to make sure the feet are far enough away from the door so that that the knee is not hyper-extending. A side view will look like the knee is slightly above a 90-degree angle. Another way to alleviate this complaint is to have the patient press her lower back against the door because some-times this relieves knee pain. Another solution is to place a band about an inch above the knees. The band will cause the glute med (one of the butt muscles) to fire, and may provide relief for the knee pain while also alleviating some other body pains.

The "bands" can be purchased on the *Perform Better* website or from *GoFit*.

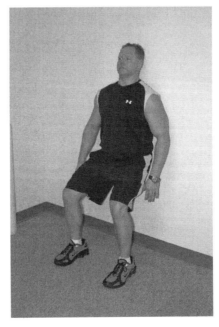

(Wall sit)

If the patient still has knee pain, try a modified version of the wall squat. When the patient has knee pain, or I believe the patient's problem is from the hip joint, I ask that the patient move the feet past shoulder width, which addresses any problem in the hip joint.

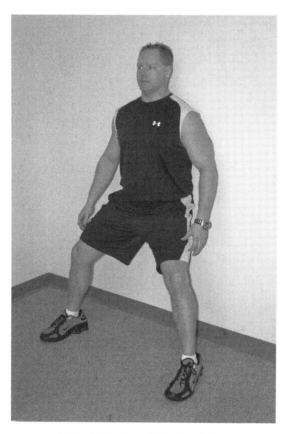

(Modified wall sit for hips)

Again, walk the feet away from the door, with the feet pointing straight ahead, but this time; have the patient squat slightly. Next, roll the hips back so that the patient's back is very flat against the door. Squat slowly with the back flat and have the patient push her knees out, opening the legs like a frog. The patient continues to squat with knees apart, making sure the nose splits the toes in

79

an even squat. Some patients slide one way or the other; towards the left or right. Correct their form so that they squat evenly and deeply. The patient's buttocks should be almost on the floor and the knees should be spread apart like a baseball catcher; with the back flat against the door, hips rolled back, and stomach sucked in.

Some of you may think the body is not designed to hold this position; however, if we look at the alimentary canal (large intestine) and the birth canal we can see this position lines up those structures to go to the bathroom or to deliver a baby. Western toilets may be chic, but humans were meant to squat to relieve themselves and in so doing, keep the hips, knees, and spine in great working order. It is rare to see knee replacements, hip replacements, and back pain where the culture can still squat deeply as seen in toddlers. Hinging at the hips vs. overstretching the knee and back, is the key to squatting properly. This exercise can help rebuild normal squatting mechanics.

CHAPTER EIGHT

The Signs of Success

How do we know that what we are doing is effective? The patient's response to the stretches and exercises will reveal the success of the effort. He will describe a number of sensations that signal success. The person does NOT have to experience all of these sensations. The things listed below are "feedbacks" to give the person awareness that an exercise selection was helpful.

1. The patient will feel taller.
2. The patient will feel lighter.
3. The patient will feel *free* or that it is easier to move.
4. The patient will sigh or take a deep breath.
5. The pain is totally gone.
6. The symptom is gone.
7. The patient feels lightheaded, woozy, weird, or cannot accurately describe how he feels other than to say he does not feel sick. Is the pain gone? If so then he is "ok". If one is uncertain then forgo any exercise or stretch that produces this feeling.
8. The patient's arms will move into the Peter Pan or Superman position, fists on hips.

9. The patient's eyebrows will lift up and his eyes will open wide.
10. The patient will smile broadly.
11. The patient will feel hot and even sweat. I do NOT want "overheated". I do NOT want panting or panicked. I do not want a flushed face or beat red or red eye balls. I am just making one aware that some people will become warm.
12. The patient's face will relax noticeably around the eyes, brow, and cheeks. You can actually see the tension leave the body.
13. The person has a BOUNCE in his step.
14. The person SPRINGS when he moves… off the floor or when walking. Springing is good.

Any of these sensations or feelings is a sign from the unconscious mind or innate wisdom. Capitalize on this success and repeat the stretches and exercises so that the patient continues to grow stronger and healthier, while feeling good and moving effortlessly.

I think children best demonstrate how we are to *move* through life. Most healthy children do these things: smile, move effortlessly, laugh, breathe deeply, and are very flexible. Usually, a child's life is spent in pain-free motion. Life is fun, exciting, joyous, effortless, liberating, and free! A corpse demonstrates the antithesis of life: still, stiff, tight, and heavy. Pain indicates we're moving away from the life position, and we need to take corrective action. We have left a state of "ease" and are now under "tension" or negative stress.

To explain this, let us look at one of the laws of physics: Suppose we draw back a pebble in a slingshot. The rubber bands of the slingshot are extremely tight. We call this *potential energy.* If our muscles are tight, energy is not being released and our potential is not being expressed. The muscles are NOT releasing, but being held in constant tension or always working. The body does not get to rest the muscles because they are always being used.

Most people have something called, "extremity dominance". The arms and legs are being used for balance vs. what they are meant to do... which is movement. For example, if someone loses his balance the arms and legs will tighten to prevent a person from falling over. The arms and legs become "hard" and "stiff". The hips and shoulders then cannot move, but instead, are stabilized preventing a fall.

Stable things do not like to move. The shoulders and hips are designed to move but the body can use the arms and legs to stabilize if necessary. Thus as we get older "grandma" cannot get her arms into her sweater or lift her arms overhead because the nervous system is using the arms as a way to balance the body to walk and move. Grandma is constantly "falling" but does not actually fall because her brain is using the arms as counterbalances to enable daily functions like walking and movement.

This is NOT effective and the arms begin to become very tight and stiff. Eventually the ability to "move" the shoulder or hip is lost and "tiny" grandma steps ensue. This does NOT happen overnight but these early "pains" and feelings of "fatigue" could be signals of poor movement patterns. Joint pain merely means there is an issue.

The exercises being employed are to free the body up to its original design. It is like breaking a bad habit, and allowing the body to heal itself by removing the interfering muscles.

We are looking for the 20% effort, and the 80% return or improvement. All the sensations above are ways to READ if one is on the right track. Some people prefer to communicate another way rather than language and feeling. For example, the person might not be able to explain or tell if one of the stretches or exercises helps. What to do? Read body language instead, in particular the face.

I say this because to use the methods in the following chapters will help improve communication and improve results. If a person moves SLOWER after a stretch or exercise, DUMP IT! A person's movement should be EASIER and QUICKER after an exercise or stretch.

Toddlers and puppies have LOTS of energy and can run... all day, and they are FAST. Some elderly people move fast too, and they move well. But other elderly people move slowly and are "slowing down". LOOK for the things that make people smile, relax and move faster. **The face/body expression or the movement (fast or slow), or the VAS pain scale (0–10), are three tools to use to evaluate the effectiveness of any exercise selection.**

The treatments administered to patients should improve their quality of life. By defining quality of life, we then can evaluate whether our treatments and methods of care are productive. Quality of life is based upon ease of movement. The easier it is to move the higher the metabolism and the less energy it requires to live. If muscles are constantly tight the body is drawing energy constantly. Tight muscles drain energy and result in fatigue.

A word of caution is necessary here. It is very important to understand what to look for to know whether you are getting the right results. You also need to be prepared for patients who want to kiss you, who want to dance, and for those who think they are *totally healed*. The patient is thrilled to be pain-free, but he also needs to understand that the pain may return because the body is not stable enough to maintain the adjustment that has been made. This is imperative because some patients will later think they are worse when the pain returns.

The fact is, the patient got relief but the body is not stable enough to hold the adjustment that brought about that relief. When people are in PAIN they cannot think clearly or SEE the BIG PICTURE.

Someone might have severe pain for 24/7 for a week and it is now gone... 'Aahh', total relief and *heaven* but one hour later back in *hell* then... the person's brain might interpret it as worse. The person fails to see ONE HOUR of relief vs. NO RELIEF.

If you had severe pain and then it was gone for an hour, but later the pain returned; you might think your condition has worsened. Why? The answer is accommodation.

We can accommodate, or get used to, living in pain. If we take the pain away, the patient is happy, but when it comes back he is looking for someone to blame. **Be sure to inform the patient that the pain sometimes returns.** Patients who do not stabilize will need support. This patient may need a *triple-pull* back brace until the body stabilizes, or a *trochanteric belt*, which may be purchased online at *Serola Biomechanics*.

A triple-pull brace is the famous "low-back brace" that can be ordered from a Chiropractor or other healthcare professional. Triple-pull because it (1) wraps around the waist to fasten, (one pull), (2) wraps to the left, the second pull and then, (3) a final wrap, or the third pull.

Let's review just a few of my patient's complaints and the subsequent treatment plans. Remember it is very important to observe the patient and listen closely to what he tells you. For example, I had a patient who looked like his pelvis was totally shifted to the right and his shoulders and upper body were going to the left. He was in agony. In fact, he could barely put his left foot on the ground due to severe sciatica pain.

The patient had been living like this for nine months. He went to work every day but did not get much work done. He drove an old car that did not have power steering; the springs in the seat were shot. In summary, he suffered from intractable pain with a severe antalgic lean, or leaning sideways.

Before we can determine how to help this man, we first must understand why his body is distorted this way. The first thing I did was to have him do *McKenzie* lateral pelvic deviation work with his left leg positioned behind him. This patient noted the outside part of his leg was burning. I thought to myself, "What is in that area and what burns?" I concluded that his left IT band was involved and the antalgia occurred as the body's response to relieve a lateral disc protrusion or herniation. His body was telling me what to do. **I just duplicated his body's innate wisdom**, and pushed more to the left and stretched the IT band.

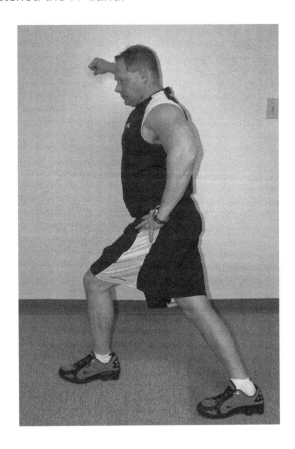

As soon as I did what the body wanted to do, this man's pain dropped in half. Nine months of pain relieved in just a few minutes. I now had an understanding of his problem and could develop a plan to restore him to wellness. Today he is like new. We relieved his pain and stabilized his condition, and then we strengthened his weak muscles and taught him how to lift properly. Relieving pain is just the first step in helping the patient experience wellness. Exercise and education are necessary to prevent a recurrence of the disabling problem that first brought the patient to the office.

Another case study involves a woman who was bent forward at the waist. She suffered from extreme neck and low back pain. Her legs were hyper-extended and her neck was so tight that it twisted to one side, resulting in torticollis (a condition where the neck muscles are in extreme spasm and the patient is unable to turn the head without severe pain). Why? Upon examination, I determined that her body was either trying to activate the hamstrings to return normal balance, trying to activate the abs, or trying to activate both the hamstrings and abs to return normal motion. Her neck was tight because she was using her neck muscles instead of her diaphragm to breathe. Why? The abs are antagonistic muscles of the diaphragm. If the diaphragm cannot contract fully because of weak abs, then the accessory muscles (neck muscles) have to compensate.

Her hamstrings were tight so we stretched them to see if that helped. **Her body was already trying to do that anyway, so we did what the body wanted to do.** If stretching does not work, then activating the hamstrings could help since this is also what the body seems to be trying to do. Maybe the body wants to do both; stretch and activate or activate then stretch. When I do not know what to do, I just stretch and see what happens. Typically, when someone is in very bad shape, stretching works best.

Remember, listen to the patient, observe what the body is doing, and then try to replicate what the body wants to do. In this particular case, I used an exercise to activate her stomach muscles and I also had her do some stretches for her hamstrings. After doing these two things, her neck pain improved. **As I tell many patients, I really don't know what to do, but the patient's body does.** I simply observe the patient's body movements to determine if what I am doing is making her better or worse. A patient that moves better informs us that we did the right thing. A patient who moves slower or has increased pain is indicative of a path we should abandon.

A common complaint that brings a new patient into the office is low-back pain that decreases with movement but is typically worse in the morning. Most of the other maladies that people suffer stem from this problem as well. The low back is the foundation and if the foundation goes, so does everything else. Let's review another case study of a gentleman who was in extreme pain from just this problem. It was very uncomfortable for him to sit down. In the standing position, his belt was pointing toward the floor. He was very guarded, tense, and was constantly on the move. Based on these observations, I determined that he wanted to move and his pelvis was rotated anterior because his belt pointed toward the floor. I needed to figure out what to do to help alleviate his pain. I always follow the three commandments:

1. **Never create or reproduce the symptoms that brought the patient into the office!**
2. **Always respect the Great Physician!**
3. **Always use perfect form and technique.**

I had him perform wall sits/air chair and that one exercise relieved about half of his pain. After doing the wall sits/air chair the patient was able to sit down and then lie down on the table. He needed to bend his knees while lying on his back, which was just fine with me. I wanted to get him supine so I could start the MEB 3 evalua-tion/treatment. Remember, these stretches are designed to unlock the pelvis/core. During the MEB 3 protocol we found that he had extremely contracted hip flexors/psoas. Remember that he had an anterior pelvis? The reason was his tight hip flexors, which is the main culprit in an anterior rotated pelvis.

The wall sits/air chair and PNF of the hip flexor group helped to identify his problem and alleviate a majority of his pain in one office visit. I just kept repeating the same movements. The patient stayed in the wall sits/air chair position until he felt as though his legs were *on fire*. I observed that the longer the wall sits/air chair, the greater the relief.

STIMULUS→ RESULT (GOOD), THEN DO MORE

When the patient was in the wall sits/air chair position, he had no pain. That is a key to treating patients. Put the patient in a position, or have the patient perform an exercise that reduces or eliminates pain and then repeat, repeat, and repeat. Do more reps or hold the position as long as possible. This works most of the time as long as we are not violating the commandments.

As soon as I identified the movements or positions that decreased his pain, I was able to develop a plan to eliminate his pain (symp-toms). The Great Physician within the patient revealed what to do and how to get my patient moving in the right direction. I quickly identified two exercises that were effective for this patient. Then the patient repeated those exercises until either the pain level reached a 3 on a scale of 1 to 10, or until it did not work any longer, or the patient reached a plateau.

If you find something that works well, then stay with it. Those two exercises, PNF of the psoas and wall sits/air chair, work extremely well for patients who present with low-back pain that feels better

89

when they are moving. This pattern also works extremely well for patients with sciatica. You will need to be careful getting the patient into the hip flexor stretch position, but once the patient can do it, immediate relief often follows. If the patient cannot get into the hip flexor stretch, then we do some modified versions of this stretch. My philosophy is that there is more than one way to achieve a particular result. In other words, let us stretch the hip flexors via a different method.

The key is to do what works best and fast. Let us not forget who is the doctor; the internal *doctor* within the patient. Remember that the patient's internal wisdom knows best and knows a lot more than we do. Observe what is working for the patient. The tools I give you are just that: tools. Try a tool to see if it works for the patient. If the "tool" or "exercise" is not EFFECTIVE then we need to do something else because we are violating the 80/20 principle. It is NOT working so… move on.

On a side note, we have to move past your fear and the patient's fear. Some people will say "no" not because it hurts, but because they are afraid. There could be a really sound reason why the patient is fearful, or it could be misplaced, irrational fear. We have to find the answer as to what will really help the patient or risk doing something that could irritate the issue. We need to determine whether what we propose to do will be effective. **My best advice is to try a <u>gentle, minimal stretch</u> or exercise and then assess the patient's response.** Is the stretch or exercise creating pain relief, or an increase of joint pain or nerve pain? **Muscle pain or muscle stretching is fine. Nerve pain and joint pain are a not.**

In an attempt to determine how much of a stretch or exercise to do, think about walking across an ice-covered lake. A wise person would not stomp boldly onto the ice in an attempt to cross the frozen lake. Instead he would step carefully onto the ice to see if it is soft or makes a noise like it is about to crack. Only if it was safe would he proceed.

Similarly, apply only enough stimuli to observe the patient's response to them. Is the patient's condition improving or getting worse? Stay calm and remain objective in your interaction with the patient. Did it help or did it make it worse? If it is worse, then do the exact opposite motion, or use some of the other tools I provide. If the patient is in very bad shape and muscle activation is not working, then go to stretching exercises. Sometimes we need a combination of both, and other times we need to be weighted more on just stretching or just muscle activation/exercises.

CHAPTER NINE
SOLUTIONS FOR PERPLEXING SCENARIOS
"I DON'T KNOW WHAT TO DO..."

Let me reiterate the purpose for this book: it was written to address the most difficult challenges a patient presents and provide solutions for your most perplexing scenarios. This book is not about correcting the underlying problem. The focus here is on alleviating the patient's pain as quickly as possible, so that the underlying problems may be identified and corrected over a period of time. The goal is to make exercises and stretches simple and safe, which in turn generates a predictable outcome.

It is very important that you closely observe all patients as they attempt to do these exercises and stretches. Some patients do not acknowledge the severity of the pain they are in because they have a hardcore mentality that refuses to accept weakness, so they ignore or deny it. If the patient feels a sensation in the area of pain and/or cannot quantify whether it is better or worse, then stop the exercise. Why? These patients have a mentality to do what they are asked to do, no matter what. In so doing, they cause harm to themselves. Be cautious with these patients as they attempt the exercises and stretches that follow.

A second group of patients just does not understand. They are not really connected or at all aware of their body. These patients have learned to suppress their feelings and it is very difficult for them to answer questions. They try to help you by responding that they think they are feeling better, or they simply say they do not know. Again, it is important to stop doing anything until these patients understand what hurts them, what helps them, and that they are in charge of determining what to do. If they do not understand, then you must learn to read their facial expressions and body language as they attempt the exercises and stretches that follow.

Legs over a Chair/Static Back is a neutral and relaxing pose. Most patients know this one innately. Static back occurs when the back goes out and the patient lies on the floor with his legs over the seat of a chair or the arm of a couch. **This is static back exercise, which works well for low-back, mid-back, shoulder, neck, and you-name-it pain**. The patient should stay in this position until the back is flat on the floor or table. If pain increases after the patient is in that position, then it is time to get up. Some patients will have a hard time getting into this position. If raising the leg increases the patient's pain, then you will need to lift the patient's legs for him.

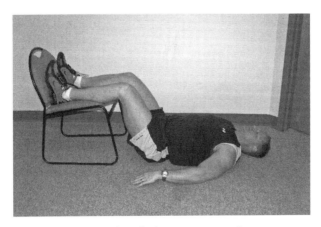

(Static back/legs over a chair)

Close observation may reveal that the patient is holding his breath. Make sure you remind the patient to breathe because many patients who are in severe pain stop breathing. Holding the breath increases pain by increasing intrathecal pressure, which is pressure around the central nervous system; e.g., brain, disc, nerves, much like *Valsava's test,* which is used to determine whether the patient has a herniated disc or pinched nerves.

If the patient cannot lie on the table, you might want to PNF the hip flexors, followed by wall sits/air chair because when raising the leg increases low-back pain or sciatica pain, it usually indicates a hip flexor contracture.

Seated glute med activation is a stabilizing exercise that is highly effective in reducing pain. Have the patient sit with the legs about hip width apart and with his feet flat on the floor. Now place your legs on the outside of his legs or use a small band by *GoFit* or *Perform Better.* (Let the patient know that you are coming into their personal space.) Have the patient external rotate or push out the legs against your legs. Make sure the patient pushes out hard and that he continues to push. Check the patient's level of pain. Most pain in the neck, low-back, shoulder, wrist, elbow, and knee will go away. This one exercise will relieve the pain and the patient will wonder how it happened.

If this helps then the person in pain can place his hands on the outside of the knees and apply pressure as he pushes outward. The picture shows me standing so that the band can be seen but we want the patient sitting.

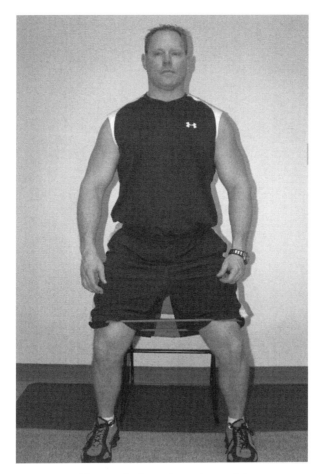

(Seated glute band meds)

The glute med stabilizes the SI joints, the body's foundation, and many a problem is due to an unstable pelvis. The glute med stabilizes the legs and prevents the legs from bowing in during walking and squatting motions, thus eliminating knee pain. The glute med stabilizes the SI joint and eliminates low-back pain and sciatica. The glute med needs to activate to stabilize the SI joint to enable lifting of the arms, which requires shoulder stability. The glutes also move CSF fluid to the brain and, as a result, can eliminate headaches and neck pain.

If you are ever uncertain or confused about how to help your patient, try the seated glute meds exercise. Most people get instant relief from it. Any time one of the protocols for neck, shoulder, knee, low-back, or headaches isn't going as well as you like, do this exercise.

Low-back Pain and/or Sciatica

Low-back pain and sciatica are very difficult to treat. Here is what to do for the worst-case scenarios when the patient is scared and in severe pain. Observe the patient very carefully. Listen closely as the patient tells you what makes him feel better or worse. Observe the patient's behavior and posture. Is the patient bent forward, to the side, or leaning back? Stand back, think about it, and then apply some of the methods that replicate what the body wants to do. Try wall sits/air chair first, because it is very effective most of the time. If the patient does not get any relief, then go after the psoas next. Strike two? Then go after the glutes. Remember: if one stretch or exercise makes the muscle group feel worse, try the exact opposite motion to see if that improves the condition. Most of the time it will! Stick to the commandments to achieve miraculous results.

Start with the MEB 3 protocols of stretching and muscle activation. The psoas stretch and erector stretch relieve pain quickly. If the patient cannot get on the table, start with wall sits/air chair. If the patient lies down and gets spasms, then get her up and do wall sits/air chair. Why? Because lying down is making it worse. Observe the patient's body language and facial expressions to be sure that what the patient verbalizes gives you a clear picture of the patient's condition. If the patient politely attempts to do as the doctor says, it will not help the patient or the doctor.

Note: You do not have to attempt everything listed in any protocol in this book. I have provided a set of tools; it is up to you to determine which of these tools will benefit your patient. You will find something that works if the exercise or stretch is done correctly. It is very important that you use just one or two tools at a time, because you do not want to get ahead of the body's healing curve. If you introduce too many new movements, the patient could actually get worse.

STIMULUS→RESULT = GOOD → REPEAT STIMULUS/(EXERCISE OR STRETCH)

STIMULUS→RESULT = BAD→ STOP→INVERSE OR DO OPPOSITE MOTION OR RETURN TO WHAT WORKED

Wall sits/Air chair. This exercise was discussed earlier in the MEB 3 protocol but needs to be mentioned again. This is one of the most predictable methods or techniques to use to eliminate severe back spasms and pain. This exercise also relieves many other problems like neck and shoulder pain.

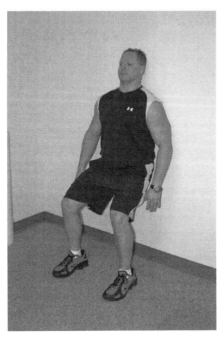

(Wall sits or air chair)

PNF of the psoas. The person will lie on his back at the edge of a table, bench or bed and bring both knees to the chest and hold them with one's hands. Then SLOWLY let one leg fall towards the floor. Apply "gentle" pressure on the leg that is dangling towards the floor. Next have the person attempt to raise the leg up against about 10-20% resistance. The leg does not move up. In other words, the leg is remaining still but the person is merely contracting the muscle just a little bit as the person doing the stretching is providing some resistance. This is not a muscle strength contest between the stretcher and patient.

After the person contracts the muscle for about 30 seconds with about a 20% effort instruct the person to relax. What one should observe is that the leg relaxes more and the leg falls more towards the floor, an increased range of motion.

Now that the leg has dropped down the "stretcher" will press down or stretch the muscle some more. Be gentle. After 30 seconds of stretching have the person attempt to raise the knee towards the chest at about 20-50% effort. The person doing the stretching prevents movement of the leg. Do this for about 10-30 seconds. Then do one final stretch to the muscle as noted above.

So... it is knees to chest. The person allows the leg to drop to the floor. The stretcher asks the person to raise the leg with 20-50% effort for 30 seconds. The person then relaxes and the stretcher applies slight downward pressure for 30 seconds. At the "new" position, the patient's leg is more towards the floor; the stretcher applies the 20-50% resistance or stretch again.

What can be expected or what will the patient feel after the stretch upon standing? The patient will most likely feel woozy or dizzy after this stretch and his pelvis will feel like it is where it needs to be. Many patients will wiggle or dance after this stretch. A patient who is in serious pain will not. He will sigh or his facial tension will relax. Many people feel taller after the stretch.

Stay within the framework of the *Miracles in Minutes* System... the stretch is alleviating the pain and "helps". Stop if the person is getting more pain. Be gentle... quantify the pain, for example a 6/10 for low-back pain. Now do the stretch. If the pain goes to a 7/10 on the pain scale then stop the stretch. If the pain goes to a 4/10 then the psoas stretch is helping.

The stretches are SUGGESTIONS that typically work for certain conditions but... we have to do what works for the particular individual in front of us. Assume nothing, and be open to everything. Set the baseline, then proceed.

Some people will feel great but then after standing for a couple of minutes the pain comes back. If the pain keeps coming back, then the person might need a back brace to stabilize and allow the stretch to take effect.

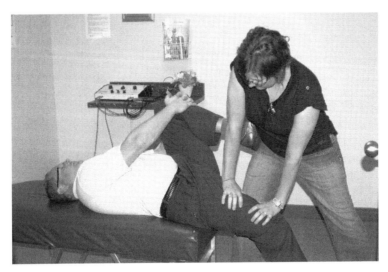

(Psoas Stretch)

Seated or lying band glute meds. Place a resistance band above the patient's knees while he is in a sitting position, then have her abduct (spread apart the legs) with the band on. The patient can do this exercise lying on one's back or sitting. If the person cannot sit, then do it lying down while they have their legs over a chair or doing static back..

If it works really well, then encourage the patient to purchase a band for use at home or while sitting at a desk at work. The patient should perform this exercise for one–two minutes at a time, and then take off the band and rest. The patient can repeat this exercise once or twice an hour if his pain is very intense and this method helps.

Do the "relieving exercise" one or two times an hour or as needed.

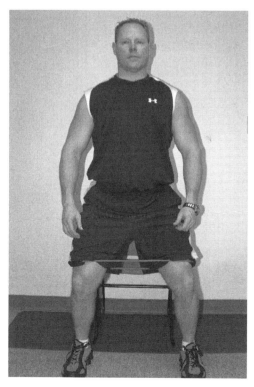

(Seated glut band meds)

Prone over table single leg raise (Cox position). Have the patient place his trunk on the table with his legs resting on the ground. Make sure the patient is comfortable. The patient's low-back/leg angle will be about 45 degrees. The patient initiates the movement by first squeezing the glutes (butt muscles). After glute activation has occurred, the patient raises the leg and holds. The person is not permitted to lift the leg if he cannot activate the glute.

You may have to goad, dig, or touch the patient to make him aware of the glute. The glute is the first thing that should fire upon extension of the leg to stabilize the hip joint. If the glute does not fire, then the hip will move into anterior femoral glide causing pelvic and lumbar instability.

Anterior femoral glide is something described by Shirley Sarhmann, PT. Basically the hip is banging the heck out of the socket and grinding the hip away. The body compensates by making the lower back unstable and unstable joints are PAINFUL joints. *The back hurts but the hip might be the culprit or the cause of the back pain.*

This exercise is not done as a set of reps, down and up, down and up. This exercise is just lift, and hold for a time. As the patient is doing the exercise, check his pain level. Is it getting better or getting worse? If the pain is reduced, continue the exercise. If lifting one leg makes the pain worse, then try the other leg. If either leg does not help alleviate the pain then STOP. We are looking for that 20% effort with 80% return. An exercise that cuts the pain in half is the exercise of choice. *I cannot stress this enough.*

Be observant... it seems logical if we do an exercise to one leg we should do it on the other side too. DO NOT assume anything. For example, raising the left leg improves the back pain and as soon as the right leg is being exercised the pain shoots up. Stop doing the right leg and ONLY DO the left leg because the left leg alleviated the pain as described in this scenario. If both sides help, then do both sides. If neither works, then DUMP the exercise. We are NOT doing work or exercise for the sake of exercise. The *Miracles in Minutes* System is a result driven method… we only do what works or helps in the 80/20 method.

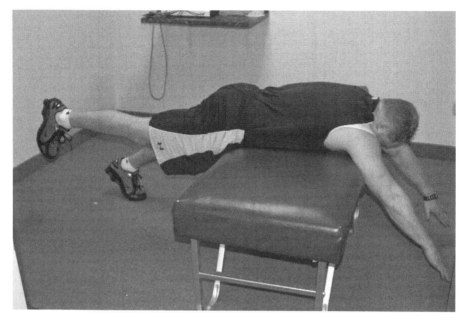

(Prone single leg raise)

If ever you do something that increases the patient's pain, stop, and go back to what worked and repeat it. It is a simple balancing equation. If what you do alleviates 50% of the patient's pain, then leave it alone until the next visit.

Some people who have very low energy or severe pain might be able to do only one or two exercises. We are NOT seeking to find as many exercises as possible. The GOAL is to find the exercise or stretch that produces the "miracle relief"… whatever that may be.

If you can find only one thing, a stretch, or activation, then do that. Focus on doing what works at that moment, especially for patients with low energy or severe pain. You can try other stretches and exercises later as the patient's pain threshold is lowered. Be patient… doing *more* is NOT always *better*. As soon as the person has decent relief such as 50% relief then call it a day.

Janda sit-ups. A Janda sit-up is done by digging the heels into the ground or bracing the back of the leg against the table. This is a surprising quick remedy that can alleviate low-back pain. Sit the patient on the edge of the table and then ask him to try to crunch forward.

If a patient with low-back pain presents with forward antalgia, leaning over at the waist, then the body might be trying to activate the abs. The person is bent over for a reason will continuing to bend forward alleviate or fix the issue?

The *Janda sit-up* is named after a famous world expert on low-back pain. Janda, a Czech neurologist, noted that by activating the glutes/hamstrings, the body would inhibit the hip flexor group.

It is theorized that overactive "hip flexors" such as the psoas cause many low-back pains and disc herniation. So the Janda sit-up is utilized to have the hip flexor release or turn off and in doing so for some people the "back pain" goes away.

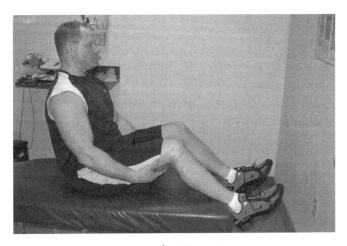

(Janda Sit-up)

McKenzie lateral maneuver (left/right). This exercise is great for the people who look like the Leaning Tower of Pisa. We can also use this exercise for lateral leg pain in the area of the IT band. If the patient's hips are out to the left, then push them out there a little farther. Do not forget the rule. **Do a little bit, but quickly ask, "Is it getting better or worse?"** If the pain is subsiding rapidly, then stay with this exercise.

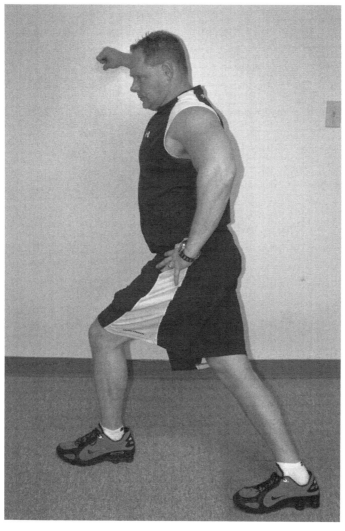

(McKenzie lateral lean)

Have the patient stand an elbow's length away from the wall and place the leg closest to the wall behind the other leg. Now have the patient lean toward the wall. Again, ask if the pain is getting better or getting worse. How much relief did the patient get: 30 percent, 50 percent, or 70 percent? Remember the premise of this book is to find the exercise or exercises that pay a handsome reward quickly. If the person gets a huge dividend, say 70 percent relief, then I would invest in that exercise repeatedly.

Standing toes out glute squeeze. This exercise helps to relieve low-back pain, and is also a good way to relieve knee, neck, and hip pain. The BIG PICTURE is that the body is a system and pain or injury is not a single-area condition. Muscles connect to muscles. I highly recommend reading Tom Myers's book, *Anatomy Trains* to really grasp the concept.

Have the patient stand with his feet pointed out at 45-degree angles and then squeeze and release his gluts tightly. Squeeze and release. Squeeze and release. This exercise will help the glutes stabilize the pelvis. This exercise is very different from the band glute meds.

If the patient cannot do this while standing, then have him try it lying on his stomach or back. Remember, the rule is to get the patient into a comfortable position and then try to get the stabilizing muscles to work again. Pain means the body is unstable.

Erector spinae stretch/lateral line stretch. This stretch is part of the MEB 3 protocol for all problems, but it warrants a mention in this section because this stretch relieves pain fast. Pay special attention to details in doing the stretch. If the person cannot tolerate both sides, then only do one side. Only do what works or helps. Observe the results… the person is feeling better or the person is feeling worse. We CANNOT assume that doing the other side will help as well. It may… it may not.

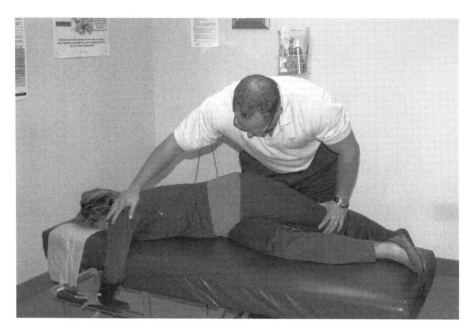

(Lateral Line Stretch)

Quadruped shoulder blade squeeze. This exercise is also great for headaches, shoulder pain, low-back pain and neck pain. If possible, have the patient get on the floor on his hands and knees. Babies learned to crawl this way and crawling prepared the body for walking. Have the patient allow an arch to come into their back and slowly let the shoulder blades come together. Also, allow the hips to move slightly in front of the knees. Again, while doing this exercise we want to make sure the body is in alignment.

Remember proper alignment: ankle, knee, hip, and shoulder are lined up and the pelvis and shoulders are level with the floor. If we want to realign the body, then we have to put the body into that position. However, do not force things into place.

Simply get into the position and the person needs to merely relax. By relaxing the person stops "struggling" with himself and the body automatically knows how to heal itself. The person ALLOWS the change to take place vs. "forcing the issue".

Again, check with the patient and listen to what his internal doctor is telling him. If the patient is okay and the pain is getting better, just keep him in this position. What is the rule? Keep a patient in a position if the position results in the patient's pain being reduced. Whatever position, stretch, posture or exercise that produces the *Miracle in Minutes* is the correct selection, keeping in mind the 20% effort that produces the 80% result.

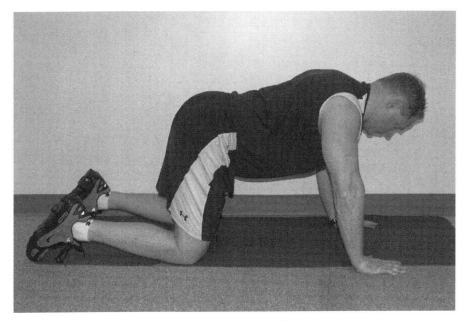

(Quadruped, or on all fours)

Standing table. This stretch will look familiar to you if you do Yoga. Ask the patient to stand with his feet hip-width apart, facing a table, counter top, or the back of a chair. The patient should then bend over so that his hips move backward and his arms rest on the table, counter top, or the back of the chair. The body should look like an "L". The bottom of the "L" is the feet on the floor and the top of the "L" is the hands on the counter. The patient has just moved through the hip axis, creating greater motion. To increase the effects of the stretch, relax the upper body allowing the chest to move toward the ground, which allows the spine to move through its full range of motion.

What I've done is identify which exercises and stretches are most helpful in alleviating pain caused by particular injuries.

People tend to exercise without giving thought to what they are doing. They just do it without noticing if the exercise or stretch is improving their health. As a result, they do some good and some bad, but often leave the gym or Yoga class feeling worse. Then they conclude that exercise is bad for them. Exercise in itself is not bad, but an exercise done the wrong way, or at the wrong time might be too much for a body that is out of alignment. The stretches and exercises in this book are to be used only if the simple rule is followed: **do what helps the patient.** Do not do anything that makes the patient's complaint worse.

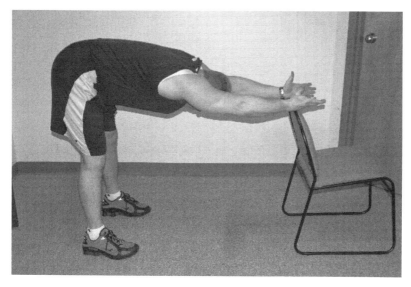

(Standing "L" or tabletop)

Glute bridge. This is one of my favorite exercises because it helps to keep the pelvis in its proper alignment by engaging the hamstrings and glutes. First, do some psoas work with the patient so that the pelvis can move into its proper position by getting the shortened hip flexors out of the way. One may not be able to do the glute bridge exercise if the person is in intractable pain.

Have the patient lie on her back on the floor or table, with knees bent. Ask the patient to slowly lift her buttocks off the floor, but be sure the patient does not experience low-back pain as a result of this movement. Next, the patient should lift her toes up and drive her heels into the floor, which activates the glute max. When the hips, shoulders, and knees are in a straight line the patient has good form. If the glute does not fire properly, the patient will have low-back pain or a "Charlie horse" in the hamstrings. The goal is that the buttock muscles get a workout, with no back pain or cramps in the hamstring. These are "no-no's". Dump the exercise and move on or go back to what is working for the patient. **Each and every one of the exercises in this book is a SUGGESTION to "what" might help.** Do what works or achieves the 20% exercise with the 80% benefit.

You can also put an exercise band around the patient's knees and have the patient do this exercise for reps, down and up. Have the patient who is wearing the band slightly push the knees out and squeeze the butt muscles while lifting the buttocks off the floor. Again, raise the toes and drive the heels into the floor.

I also like isometric holds, which is when the patient just lifts up and stays there without moving. Have the patient hold the position as long as possible with good form. If the form breaks, the patient needs to stop. If a patient is experiencing low-back pain, have her drop down or; in other words, do not lift the buttocks up so high. Have the patient drop the buttocks down until the pain is gone and then hold that position.

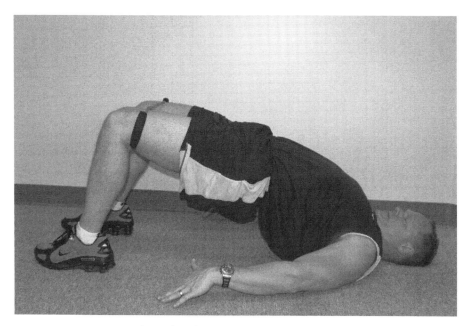

(Glute bridge shown with a band)

Quad Stretch. Have the patient place his leg behind him up on a table or kitchen counter. If the patient has bad knees, start with a low stimulus (18 inches) and then progress up to about 42 inches after several months. If the person's knees are not bad, or the back is not too bad then go right to 42 inches.

Caution: some people might get a hamstring cramp or "Charlie Horse" at the higher heights. Solution... put the foot on a lower surface like a chair or foot stool. If the person keeps cramping then STOP the exercise and move on. **We are going for the RESULT... pain relief of 50% or greater, and NOT the exercise or stretch.**

This stretch will help with low-back pain, headaches, knee pain, shoulder pain, stuffy noses, coughs, and neck pain. Many patients will have the knee out to the side to start, which is okay. After holding this position for 30 to 60 seconds, have the person squeeze the butt muscle on the leg being stretched. This will increase the stretch greatly and protect the back. If the back hurts, then decrease the height or instruct the patient to squeeze the buttocks. Hold the position for one to three minutes per side, and then do the other side. Repeat for low-back pain, headaches, knee pain, IT band pain, shoulder pain and most other pains. If you do not know what to do, often this stretch eliminates many pains. Back pain is a sign of doing the stretch incorrectly via too much stimuli (the leg is too high and the thigh muscles are too tight) or not squeezing the buttocks. If it is NOT working then of course... stop.

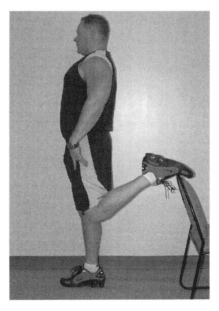

(Quad Stretch)

Supine Psoas Strengthening. Have the patient lie on his back and bring his knee up to his chest. Do not forget to ask the patient if this movement causes pain. Next the patient ,"friend" ,doctor or therapist should place a hand on top of the patient's leg and gently apply resistance as the person attempts to pull the knee up to the same shoulder. About 20-30% effort is all that is needed. Again, this is not a test of seeing who is the strongest. We just want the muscle to activate for about 30 seconds. If this does not cause the patient any discomfort, do the exercise on the other side.

Now have the patient stand. Many patients have very little psoas strength which causes the lower three hip flexors to become super dominant. When the leg passes the belt line or 90 degrees, the psoas is the primary mover. Many patients who complain of pain around the kidney area, T10-L2, will note that the pain goes away with this exercise. A tight muscle is a weak muscle. Tightening the muscle a little more can make it release and get stronger.

This exercise might also help with: Knee pain, neck pain, shoulder pain and "asthma". The psoas connects to the diaphragm and so by stimulating it I have seen a few asthma attacks stop in a few minutes. The body is governed by REFLEXES and all we are doing is turning something ON that should be on, and turning something OFF such as a muscle that is working overtime.

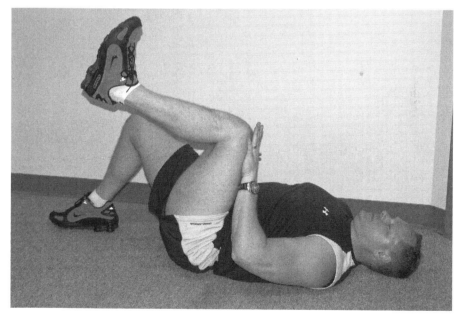

(Psoas Strengthening)

Spiderman. This stretch is not for everyone; be very cautious in doing this stretch because it will help some patients, but not all. If you are unsure or the patient seems too acute, then forgo this one. There are many other stretches and exercises already identified that can help the patient safely.

Have the patient step out into a lunge at 2 o'clock position as far as can be tolerated, which means the right leg steps out to 2 as if he is looking at a big clock on the floor. Now slowly let the right arm slide down the inside of the right leg and the left arm can go to the floor for support. Stay in this position as long as the patient does not have an increase in his pain level or if the pain is reduced. Remember, the rule is to find a position that alleviates pain and then hold it. After holding this stretch for 30 seconds or so, have the patient bring the other leg up to meet the forward leg or to walk forward. Now do the other side. If the stretch worked well, then repeat it twice. If the patient has really bad balance or is having a hard time getting into the stretch then use a Swiss ball or chair to lean on.

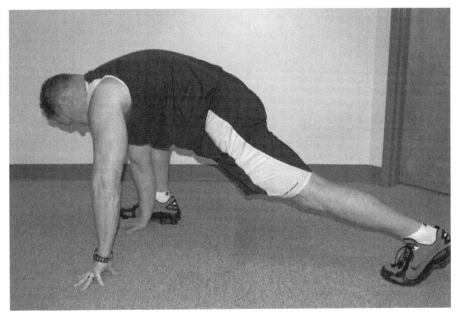

(Spiderman)

Sumo squat walk. If Spiderman has worked well, then the patient will benefit from this exercise. First, ask the patient to turn his feet out to the 45-degree-angle position, then have him squat down and walk in this position. The Sumo Squat Walk opens up the hip joints and helps to restore functional mobility very quickly. **If the patient has severe knee pain do not do this exercise.** Instead, do the quad/rectus femoris stretch.

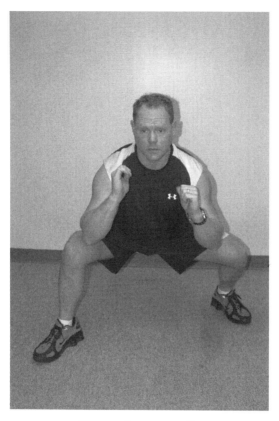

(Sumo Squat Walk)

Horse Stance. The Chinese say, "A man is only as strong as his horse." Most martial arts movements are built upon "horse stance" and the better at the stance, the better the martial artist.

115

Man is much like a tree trunk and every tree trunk must have roots. Rooting is the ability to plant our feet into the ground and draw strength from the earth. Most people are not rooted well and to do horse stance we need to talk about rooting and how to prepare for it.

I recommend that the patient remove her shoes to "root" better into the floor. Additionally, many patients' shoes have worn unevenly, thus doing the horse stance with the shoes on will only hinder the patient's progress. The patient should stand with her feet apart, a little wider than hip-width apart. Turn the feet out slightly, bend the knees slightly, and tuck the tailbone between the legs by sucking in the stomach. While standing, get the ball of the first toe, the ball of the pinky toe and the heel to touch the ground evenly. Note the triangle formation of the three points. In geometry, the strongest shape is the triangle.

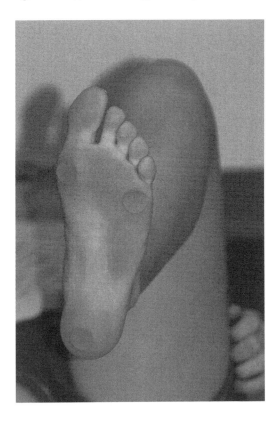

Next, have the patient screw the feet into the ground. The left foot will screw into the ground counter clockwise and the right foot will screw into the ground clockwise. Now spread the toes apart wide while screwing the feet into the ground with the three points of the foot placed evenly on the ground. There should be movement in the hip joint and the patient should feel the buttocks tighten.

Next, allow the weight to shift to the inside of the foot (along the arch) but keep the screwing movement going with the three points of the foot touching the ground. At this point, the patient will feel a lot of action happening in the buttocks.

The final step is to suck in the belly button and contract the pelvic muscles, similar to doing the Kegel exercise. Make sure the tailbone is between the legs. This activates the pelvic floor/pelvic diaphragm and makes the glutes work. This exercise stabilizes the entire body and relaxes the upper body, creating good posture and good curves.

This position is a building block for all stabilization exercises performed in the upright position. If it is done correctly the patient enjoys a feeling of power, stability, and strength. The Chinese call it "rooting." The better the tree's root system, the more able the tree is to gather nutrients, withstand strong winds, and produce fruit. The same goes for us.

Western biomechanics calls this stabilization of the hips/pelvis, sacroiliac joints, lumbosacral articulation and lumbar spine along with establishing a functional lower extremity kinetic chain. This means the spine is stable and strong, the patient has no pain and feels very powerful. This exercise if very difficult to execute, but worth the hard work of learning it because of the wonderful benefits it provides.

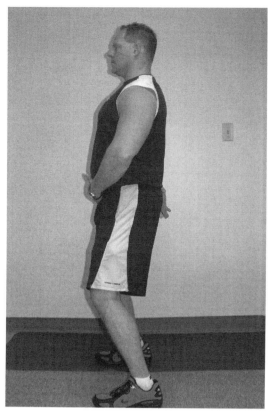

(Horse Stance)

Sorensen's Test/Hyperextension Exercise. Many low-back-pain sufferers experience immediate relief upon doing this exercise/test. Have the patient lay on her stomach across a table so that the pelvis is slightly off the table. If a person is weak or frail, move back so that more of the pelvis is on the table. Next, have the patient place her hands on the floor for support, squeeze her buttocks and slowly rise up, taking her hands off of the floor. Hold this position for time. Do not allow the patient to experience low-back pain, but only do a hyperextension first using the glutes to do the lifting, then the hamstrings.

This is not for very acute patients unless you have a good handle on it. Some acute patients will feel great immediately afterward. Fred Hatfield, known as *Dr. Squat* for his ability to squat 1,000 pounds, used a similar exercise to heal a herniated disc in his low-back. The weight lifters called this reverse hyperextensions and it works great for improving proper lifting mechanics. This exercise is not just for Dr. Squat. I also use it on a 79-year-old grandmother and her 84-year-old husband. At first, she was reluctant to do it; now that she is confident about doing it, she tells me to "get in here and do your job." She is halfway across the table before I even get in the room, and when we finish she feels great.

We are working the most powerful kinetic chain in the body—the posterior kinetic chain—which is what enables us to squat, lift, and jump.

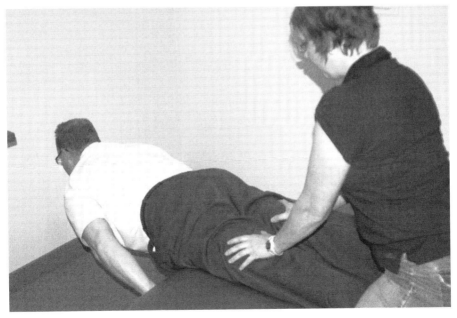

(Sorenson's Test or Hyperextension Exercise)

CHAPTER TEN

HEADACHES

Headaches are typically indicative of a decreased oxygen supply to the brain. Headaches in different areas like centralized headaches, frontal, occipital, parietal and temporal usually indicate dural tension. The tension is often due to stress and/or dehydration. Again, a lack of oxygen is the main component of headaches. Water is H_2O, two hydrogen molecules and one oxygen molecule. The patient does not drink enough water and/or holds her breath. This is the main culprit or cause of headaches.

Typically, people who have many headaches are under a lot of stress. Most headache sufferers have a coping mechanism for stress that actually causes the headache. When frightened, angry, or offended by another person or situation, the headache sufferer grits her teeth and holds her breath as a means of self-control. In an effort to be polite or respectful to someone else, she suppresses her feelings. This also occurs when she is fearful or anxious; again, she copes with the emotion by clenching the jaw or teeth. The clenching of the teeth throws off the Temporal Mandibular Joint (TMJ), which is the jawbone located right in front of the ear. This transfers stress to the Occiput/C1 vertebrae, compressing nerve structures.

On page four of the twenty-ninth edition of *Gray's Anatomy*, it is noted that compression of C1 can cause headaches.

Observe the headache sufferer and note that she holds her breath and possibly clenches her teeth during the consultation. Another sign that indicates she is stressed is that she speaks very rapidly and her eyes move rapidly, which indicates anxious thinking. Rapid conversation can put her on the verge of hyperventilating because she is breathing rapidly and not fully oxygenating the lung field or the brain.

In addition, when human beings are afraid or insecure, we tend to close our legs.

We tighten up, take a defensive position, and hold our breath. When we are angry, we grit our teeth. These are mechanisms that we use to do deal with fear and suppressed agitation, irritation, and rage. Have you ever heard someone say that she has a "raging headache?" The raging headache is nothing more than suppressed rage—at other people, life, stressful situations, and/or one's work environment. The physical manifestations of these emotional reactions are pinched nerves and stress on the nervous system.

Now that we understand why and how headaches typically occur we can help the patient get some relief. There are several tools in the following pages that will help the headache sufferer. Usually, any one of the first four stretches will do the trick. As the patient improves and the headache diminishes, a light walk and light stretching are perfect movements for the patient to do. She should not engage in any strenuous exercise because physical strain or heavy lifting will likely cause the headache to return.

Supine frogs/butterflies PNF, downward dogs, quadruped, and quad stretch are excellent tools to use to achieve headache relief.

1. **Supine frogs/butterflies PNF**. Have the person lie on his back on a table. Place the bottoms of his feet together and then let the knees fall out to the side. Gently apply pressure to the medial aspect of the knees while the patient gently resists. Ask the patient to relax and slowly stretch the legs out farther. Check with the patient during the exercise in the relax phase and active phase to see if the headache is going away. Repeat the stretch until the pain is gone. If this stretch is working, stay with it until the patient gets complete relief.

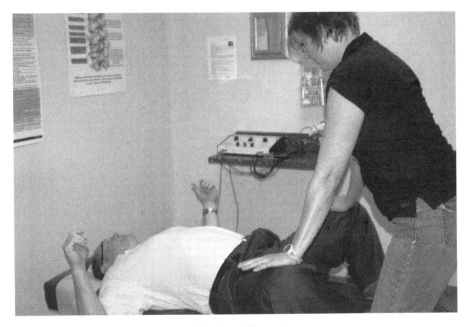

(Supine Frogs)

If you are uncomfortable doing this movement, you can substitute prone frogs instead. At times one method will be better than the other. One way is laying on one's back and the other way is facing the floor. To the brain each is a different orientation. The exercises are similar but NOT the same to the nervous system.   I prefer the supine method from a positional point of view, and because the patient is less likely to recruit the neck muscles. **Supine frog works BEST for TEMPORAL HEADACHES... headaches around the temples or above the ears. About 85% of the time this does the trick in two minutes or less!**

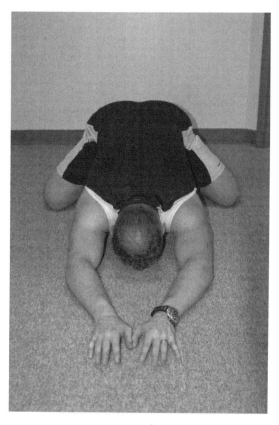

(Prone frog)

The supine frogs/butterflies PNF opened up the body and the next move or exercise is to solidify that opening. Remember, when people are frightened or agitated, they close their legs, which sometimes produces a knock-kneed effect. This is due to tight groin muscles pulling the knees together. This

124

exercise loosens the adductors to relieve the tension and release the feeling. Remember that these things occur on the subconscious level; often the patient is unaware of his body's defense mechanisms or "primal reactions" to stress.

2. **Clams or clam with a band.** I prefer clams, but the band combined with the clams or glute meds is also effective. Another alternative is for the patient to sit and do the band glute meds. Use whatever method works best for the patient. The key to doing this exercise with headache patients is to synchronize the breathing with the movements. One cause of Headaches is the patient is not breathing and typically is clenching their teeth. By breathing gently with the leg movement, the CSF pump respiratory mechanism resynchronizes and, quite often, pain disappears within minutes.

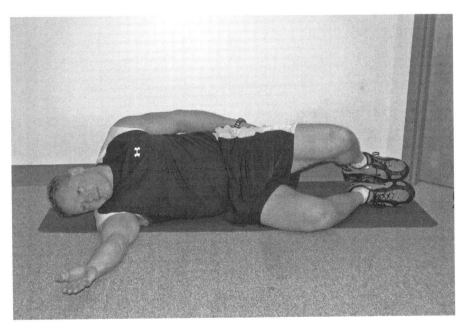

(Clams)

Have the patient lie on her side and place a pillow under the head so that there is good spinal and airway alignment. Next, have the patient abduct (spread legs) and inhale upon the opening of the legs. The patient should exhale upon closing the legs. Gentle inhale, leg up. Gentle exhale, leg down.

Please note: this is not fast breathing, but slow, gentle, relaxed breathing. By gently breathing, the patient switches into the parasympathetic nervous system allowing healing and normalization or balancing to take place. The patient is moving out of "neck breathing" into *belly breathing* or relaxed breathing.

Do not do any hard, forceful movements with headache sufferers because the headaches will become more severe and start the headache pattern up again. Forceful breathing and forceful movements increase intrathecal pressure; therefore, if a person has a headache then it is not a day for a core workout unless you really know what you are doing. It is safer to just get the headache to go away then let the patient rest.

3. **Calf Stretch.** For headaches at the back of the skull or in the forehead area do this stretch. Typically, for about 85% of people the headache is gone in less than 30 seconds, or at least, greatly reduced. Frogs and calf stretch handle most common headaches that most people are plagued with. Why wait 45 minutes for the Ibuprofen when 30 seconds can do the trick?

Stand on the edge of a step preferably at the bottom of stairwell. No need risking falling down all the stairs. Hang onto the railing or wall and allow the calf muscles to relax stretching the calf. We want the weight to shift towards the "heels" and not the toes or ball of the foot. Keep the legs straight and down and allow the buttocks to shift backwards. Ouch! Yes, most people have really tight calf muscles.

Calf stretch is also good for shoulder pain, neck pain and even low-back pain. This stretch is one of the STARS in the *Miracles in Minutes* Method.

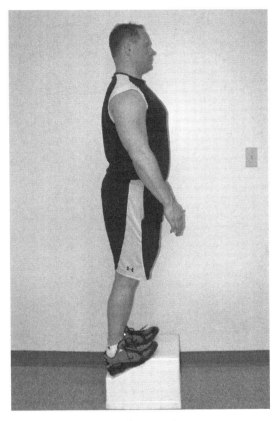

(Calf Stretch)

4. **Cats and dogs**. Many physical therapists and chiropractors call these movements *pelvic tilts*. In the practice of Yoga,

127

these positions or movements are known as *cow pose*, or *cat and dog pose*.

Part of the headache problem is improper breathing and abnormal CSF flow. Upon inhalation, the sacrum/tailbone and the occiput/skull bone move into flexion. Picture this: Inhale, hips roll forward increasing the curve in the low-back and the head or nose pushes forward, creating flexion of the occiput on C1.

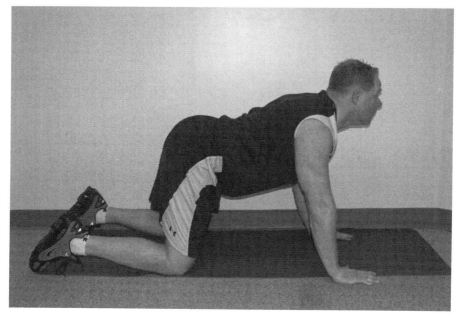

(Dog)

Exhalation is belly button sucked in while arching the back like a **scared cat**. The chin tucks toward the throat.

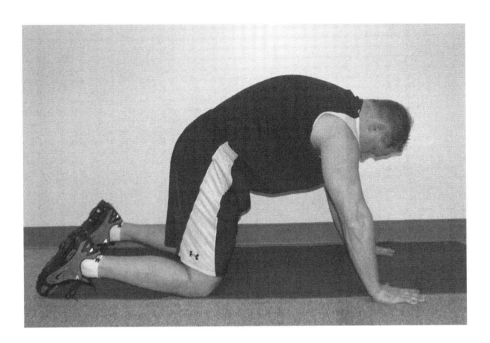

Cats and dogs, combined with inhaling upon flexion of the sacrum and exhalation upon sacral extension, are helpful in alleviating headaches. Start in the quadruped position, with the patient on his hands and knees, and allow the head and neck muscles to relax. The patient should rest in that position for a few seconds, allowing a curve to come into the lower back. Ask the patient if his headache is getting better or worse. In a majority of patients, there will be modest improvement. This position is also a great way to reduce lower back pain, shoulder pain, and neck pain.

While in the quadruped position, inhale and allow the stomach to sag while the head looks up. Gently and slowly, start to exhale while reversing the curve like a scared cat and the head looks towards the patient's feet.

The goal is not to strain, but to slowly and gently allow the body to free itself and a return to normal breathing patterns, synchronizing CSF flow with respiration. Do five cycles, or reps, and check the patient's pain level again. Please note: this is not a race to see how quickly the patient can perform this exercise.

5. **Downward facing dog.** This stretch is also taken from Yoga. One of Yoga's valuable lessons is to relax into tension. As we relax into tension, tension disappears. If we push into tension then the physical law, "every reaction creates an equal and opposite reaction," comes into play. The body pushes back to protect itself creating MORE tension.

This is a great stretch for low-back pain, hip pain, knee pain, and headaches. The stretch quickly releases dural tension, and frees up tight hamstrings and calves. Headaches and pain down the arm or leg are signs of dural tension. Poor ankle mechanics lead to poor hip mechanics, which cause all kinds of problems including sexual dysfunction. Many men who have had hip replacements have difficulty engaging in sex because hip motion is impaired. Sexual dysfunction is frequently caused by poor hip/ankle mechanics that lead to tight hips, and as I said earlier, all power or life energy is moved through the hips. In doing this simple exercise, not only can we get rid of headaches, but we can also improve the hip function.

Have the patient get into the quadruped position and straighten his legs, pushing the buttocks toward the ceiling. Most people will have a difficult time doing this and will complain about the stretching sensation. As the patient moves the buttocks toward the ceiling, have him drop his heels. Do not overdo it, but elicit enough stretch that is comfortable for the patient. Check with the patient to see if the headache pain is reduced. Make sure the patient allows his head to just fall or rest. Most people will try to raise their heads; tell them to relax their head or neck. If the patient is unable to do this stretch, or the stretch is making the headache worse, then stop.

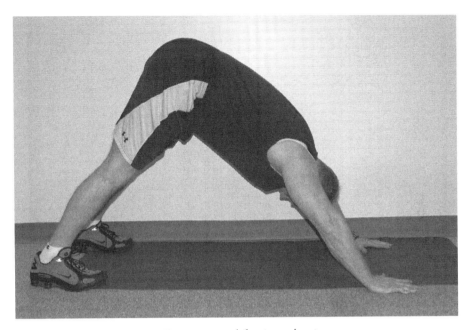

(Downward facing dog)

6. **Runner's stretch**. This stretch is great for posterior knee pain, low-back pain, sciatica, and headaches. If the patient cannot do downward facing dog, then use this stretch instead.

    Runner's stretch is similar to downward dog, but not as intense. Have the patient place one foot in front of the other, with the legs directly under the hips, and feet pointing at 12 o'clock. The patient might need to have a table or chair in front of him for balance. Next, have the patient slowly bend forward at the waist while keeping the forward leg completely straight. The patient must squeeze the quadriceps on the front leg, which lengthens the hamstring to create some muscle balance and allow the hamstring to stay lengthened.

Do this on both sides for about two minutes and as always make sure the position or stretch is not causing an increase in the patient's pain level. Frequently, the patient will note a dramatic decrease in pain.

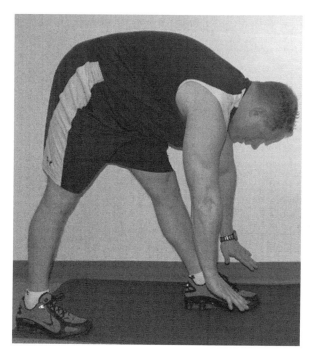

7. **Quad stretch.** This stretch is great for knee pain and for many pains besides headaches. It is one of the "magic bullets" or tools that can be thrown at a body ache or pain. For headaches at the back of the skull this works at times.

Have the patient place their leg behind them on a chair, table or counter about 42 inches high. You can also start out with a low bench or chair before moving up to the 42-inch mark. The elderly and those with severe cases will need to start with a smaller stimulus such as a chair or foot stool. Many people need something to hold on to such as a chair for balance.

Check with the patient to see if the stretch is helping. Remember the rule—only do exercises and stretches that work. If the patient is getting low-back pain, make sure the person squeezes the buttocks on the same side. Squeezing the buttocks should stop the back from hurting.

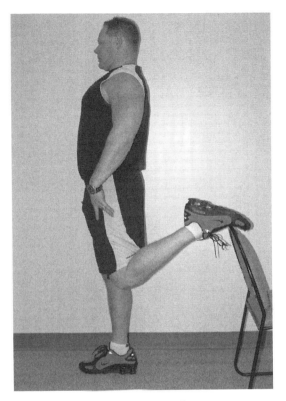

(Quad Stretch)

8. **Quadruped position.** Have the patient get down on all fours in a quadruped position. Move the hips slightly in front of the low-back. Make sure she lets her head hang down instead of trying to hold it up. Keep the arms straight. Let an arch come into the low-back, but do not force it. Now, allow the shoulder blades to come together. Is the patient feeling better? If it is making her feel worse, stop.

133

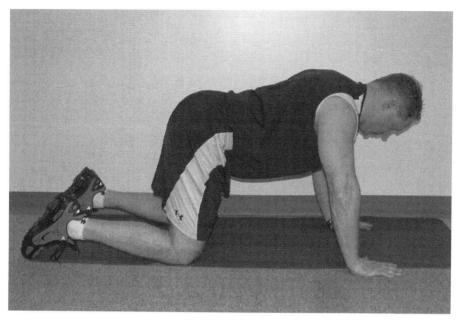

(Quadruped, or all fours)

9. **Back Brace**. A back brace for a headache? Yes, a low-back brace. Headaches, neck pain are **SYMPTOMS...** but symptoms of what? The neck is working overtime and all the muscles that support the head are being used by the body to stabilize the low-back. I know... it is "odd" but we are looking for a *Miracle* and not just the myopic... "head hurts, rub the head." The result with most of this narrow-minded thinking is "minimal."

If the patient attempted all of these stretches and nothing was effective, or the relief did not last, have her stand in front of you. Give the patient a bear hug around the hips. Did the headache go away? If the patient has **torticollis,** the neck pops right up; if the patient has a headache, she enjoys immediate relief. It is called *pelvic instability* and the patient's body has run out of compensation and needs a rest.

Torticollis: that is the nasty neck pain where the head feels like it weighs a ton. One cannot move or turn the head at all. It is EXTREMELY painful and most people get a neck brace or collar which gives only slight relief but.. the back brace.. is instant relief for many a person. Again it is "odd" or weird, but we are not limited in our *Miracles in Minutes* thinking and we are open to "anything" that provides that 80% relief with 20% effort.

One final note about how to resolve headache pain warrants some attention. I have observed that patients who have a **headache directly above the iris/eye have an ankle problem! A Chiropractic adjustment to the ankle on the side of the headache above the eye eliminates the headache in seconds. Tell your Chiropractor to adjust the talus on the same side of the headache above the eye and the headache goes away in less than two seconds.** Another method that I have found to be effective is to have the patient rotate her foot in circles until the headache goes away.

One of my patients had seen numerous neurologists and had multiple CAT scans and MRIs to determine the source of her problem. Years of suffering ended on her second visit to my office when I made the adjustment described above. Her family does not understand how the best doctors at one of the top hospitals in the world did not know how to help her.

If you suffer from various pain-related issues, you might consider seeking treatment under a chiropractor. Only a chiropractor can adjust specific segments of the body, such as the spine or another joint. If you are reading this book then you are open to new things and new ways of addressing health problems. If you are still skeptical you still might consider trying something new to see if you can find a solution to what ails you. Don't give up or *give in*, but try something else. I once heard a preacher say, "If you want something you have never had, then you have to do something that you have never done."

Chiropractors typically want their patients to be involved. We seek to move from a passive type of treatment to having our patients take an active role in their own health. A chiropractor's premise is: "motion is life, and life is motion." The lack of motion in the spine or a joint leads to joint death also known as "arthritis" and poor health. As we look at nature we can see that dead things stop moving and things that are living move. Chiropractic looks to introduce the motion to joints that have stopped moving/living and in so doing we replicate what life does... move.

There are over 150 different chiropractic techniques so a person has many choices to fit one's individual preference. There are techniques that a person hears no noise, and others where one hears a "crack". Today there are methods that use special tables, instruments, gentle movements, blocks, and too many others to list here. The point I am trying to make is at least be open to trying something that best fits your own individual needs or preference. Most chiropractors will find the best option to address your concerns, and if the doctor does not do this, then find another chiropractor. You may give up on an individual chiropractor, but don't give up on chiropractic.

Just voice your concerns to your doctor (medical or chiropractic) because, in the end, it is your LIFE and your health. No doctor can read your mind or knows what you prefer, or do not prefer. Communication is essential to results, and I am placing this TOOL TO FREEDOM upon YOU, the patient, so that YOU get the type of care you desire.

CHAPTER ELEVEN

ASTHMA

One day, a patient had an asthma attack in my office. He began to gasp and struggle for breath. I credit the Great Physician with the ideas that suddenly came to my mind. What I did to help this patient was confirmed the next day by yet another patient who began to have an asthma attack right in front of me.

The patient noted pain in the C3-C4 area (neck pain) earlier that day, which is the location of the phrenic nerve that controls the diaphragm. The diaphragm controls breathing; if the diaphragm cannot do its job, there will be a health issue somewhere in the body.

Ida Rolf, founder of *Rolfing Technique,* and Tom Meyers have expanded upon a theory that existed in the early 1900s that the body is connected through some form of *fascial web.* The latest theory in Quantum physics is called "String Theory" which states everything is connected by a string. Therefore, when we treat a part or condition we rarely—if ever—cure or heal a patient. The parts work together to support the whole.

A car is not just an engine, nor is a car just a tire. A car has an exhaust for the engine, a transmission that delivers power from the engine to the wheels, and a steering wheel to control the direction. The parts of the car serve a variety of functions that result in a driver arriving at his chosen destination.

Our bodies function in much the same way. Parts come together to support the brain, which determines whether the body operates efficiently and effectively. Pain or a health issue is one of the body's indicators that there is a problem in a part or system. If given a chance the body can repair itself!

It is up to us to figure out why the body is malfunctioning and what we can do to help it heal. Over the years I have learned that working on just one part of the body rarely produces an immediate return of healing or homeostasis. When I address the area of cause, the patient feels immediate, dramatic improvement and moves in the right direction.

When I address the symptom, often the results are poor or I wind up *chasing a rabbit*. What I mean is one thing is better and now there is a problem somewhere else. We often think it is two problems and fail to see or realize the connection of interconnected parts. We fail to see how one system affects another system.

Listed below is what I found on three separate occasions that helped my patients suffering from an asthma attack in my office. I wish I had more data or more experiences, but I list them here so that others can at least offer something to the patient or so that the patient can help his or herself. I cannot say with absolute confidence that this will work since I have only experienced this three times, but I found it pretty amazing for the patients I had the opportunity to treat.

1. **Supine frogs using PNF.** Have the patient lie on his back, placing the souls of the feet together and allowing the legs to fall out to the side. Have the patient try to close his legs as you push down—gently—to create a stretch. Have the

patient squeeze, then release, and continue to gently stretch the legs. Repeat this pattern three–seven times to get the muscles to loosen up.

Watch the patient's eyes to see if you are pushing too hard. If he winces or otherwise indicates he is in pain, stop or decrease the amount of pressure you are exerting.

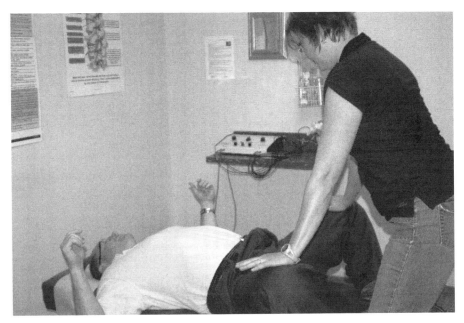

(Supine Frog)

2. **Long axis groin stretch**. With the patient still on his back, straighten out the legs. Now, take one leg and move it out to the side like a one legged jumping jack. Place your leg on the inside of the patient's leg to stretch the leg out to the side. Again, have the patient press against you and relax. In the relax phase, increase the stretch by moving the leg farther out to the side. Do this three times, holding for about 20 seconds each time. Of course do both sides, left and right, if it helps.

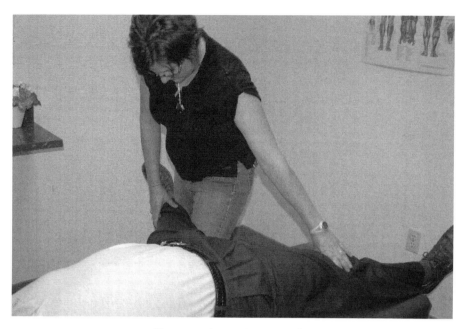

(Long axis groin stretch)

3. **Psoas activation with arms overhead**. The patient lies on his back with legs bent and feet on the table. Have the patient raise his arms above his head. Now bring the knee up to the same-side shoulder. Apply pressure to the top of the knee for resistance. Hold this for about ten seconds. Then do the other side. Check the patient's breathing. Is it better? The psoas connects to the diaphragm, so this stretch can help the diaphragm work well. Many patients use the neck and low-back to raise their legs due to a weak psoas. This exercise strengthens the psoas, so the neck and low-back can release. Therefore, this exercise can also be very beneficial for people with low-back pain, or pain around the lumbar mid-back region; especially around the kidney area.

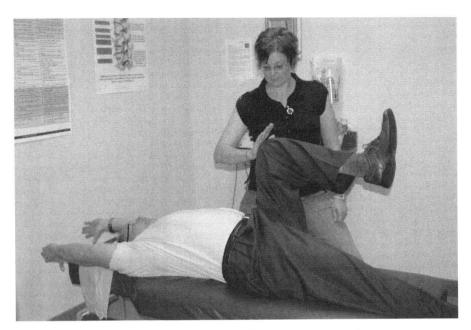

(Psoas activation with arms overhead)

4. **Side-lying clams with a band**. Have the patient lie on his side in a fetal position. Place a band around both legs and move it up to above the knees. Now have the patient raise the knee away from the other knee while the feet stay together. Inhale gently as the legs spread apart. Exhale when the leg comes down. Do 10 to 20 reps on both sides.

141

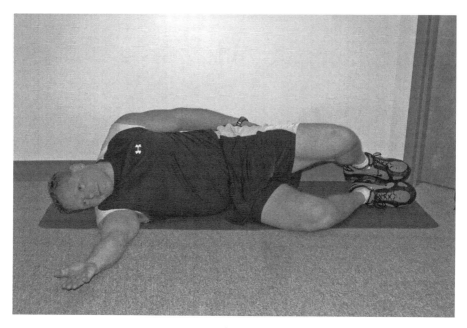

(Clams)

5. **Swimmer stretch**. Have the patient squeeze the shoulder blades together and then bend over at the waist, keeping the legs straight. Have the patient try to clasp his hands behind his back as he bends over with the thighs tight and legs straight.

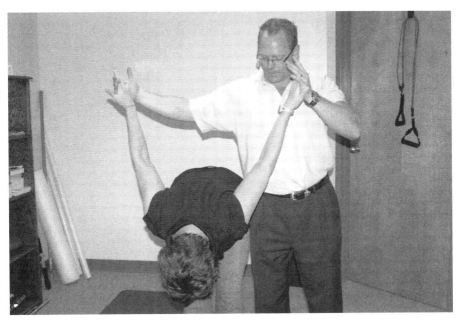

(Swimmer's Stretch)

CHAPTER TWELVE

SHOULDER PAIN

The shoulder is a very complicated joint because it is sometimes difficult to decipher the source of shoulder pain. The source of the pain may be the pelvis/hip, a shoulder position, or it could be both. I have had decent results relieving shoulder pain. One of my patients underwent physical therapy for a year, had rotator cuff surgery, and had not been able to lift her arm above her head for two years. She obtained relief in one visit, but her results are not typical.

Often shoulder pain is due to poor thoracic (mid-back or rib area) mobility due to poor pelvic (around the low-back/belt area) stability.

I have outlined some of the best exercises and stretches for the relief of shoulder pain in the next few pages. These will not stabilize the shoulder, but will provide relief from pain.

1. **Warrior I**. Have the patient step out into a lunge position with the legs in line with the shoulders. The leg that is back should feel a stretch in the front of the thigh where the leg meets the torso. The leg that is back will affect the shoulder

that hurts. The patient should be in an erect or good spinal posture position because too much trunk flexion could cause low-back pain and the stretch may not be effective.

Ask the patient to raise his arm to see if the pain improved. Many patients experience relief with this stretch because this position lengthens the psoas, which can prevent flexion of the arm, and provides the relief the person desires. Remember the arms balance out the hips and vice versa.

This method can be done standing or kneeling.

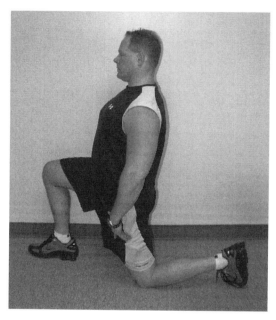

(Kneeling Warrior)

2. **Tricep kickback**. Keep the shoulder back; flex and extend the elbow. The patient is getting into a runner's position with one leg forward and one leg back. Make sure the spine is straight. The forward leg should be bent at a 90-degree-angle. Move the arm back as if he were running. Now, kick

the elbow back like a sprinter in a baton race. The patient may hold a light weight (3 lbs.).

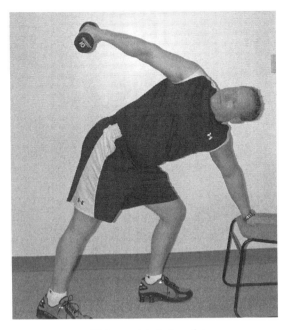

(Tricep kick back)

3. **Quad Stretch**. Have a person place his back to a table or bench. For best results, use a surface around the height of a kitchen counter. Have the patient place his leg behind him like runners do to stretch their quads. The person will feel a big stretch in the thigh muscles. While the patient is in this position ask the question, "How is your pain now?"

You could choose to do kick in the butts. All we are trying to do is stretch the quad to alleviate anterior pelvic tilt and release part of the hip flexor so that normal arm swing can return. We cannot expect the shoulder to swing out far if the hip is locked because it would throw us off balance and we would fall. Make sense now?

147

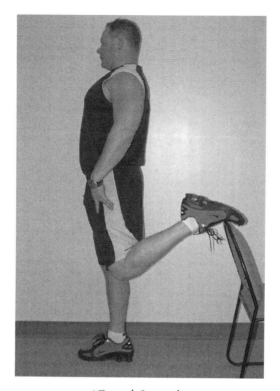

(Quad Stretch)

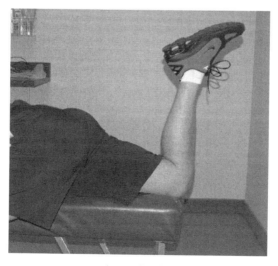

(Kick in the butts)

4. **Hamstring Stretch**. I like the Shaolin version of the hamstring stretch, or runner's stretch. The Shaolin version is to have the patient place his feet about hip-width apart. Next, bend one leg while keeping the other leg straight. Next, bend over with the torso coming down the middle of the body or nose splitting the toes while the straight leg begins to feel a big stretch. To increase the stretch, simply bend the opposite leg more and push the buttocks back creating flexion of the hip.

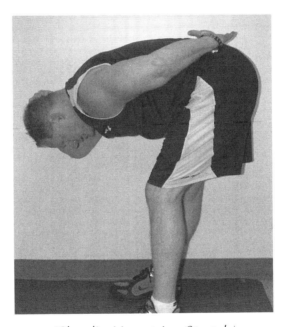

(Shaolin Hamstring Stretch)

If the "Shaolin" hamstring stretch is not helping then try the runner's stretch. Runner's stretch is to have one leg forward and one leg back while facing a table or chair. It is a lunge but both legs are straight. Now squeeze the front leg's thigh muscles (quads) and bend over, but keep the forward leg's foot on the floor with all points touching. If we are stretching the right leg, it will most likely

149

help the right shoulder. Sometimes the opposite leg will affect the opposite shoulder. The main question is… "How is your shoulder pain now in this position?"

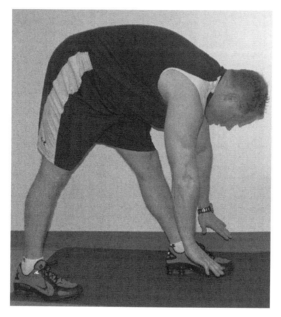

(Runner's Stretch)

5. **Upper spinal twist**. Quite often what causes shoulder pain is a lack of motion in the mid back so the scapulae (shoulder blade) wings off the body because the mid back can't move with it. Have the patient lie on his side and stack both legs on top of each other. Now allow the spine to ELONGATE, get taller or longer. Don't force it but simply breathe into the ribs sideways and the body will slowly allow the elongation. If need be, place a pillow or support under the head to allow him or her to relax. After the spine is in the elongated position, take the arm and reach back so that the knees are going one way and the arm is going the other way. The other arm should rest or hold the legs down on the ground. DO NOT

let the legs lift up or FORCE movement. Just move as much as the patient can in one day, and that is it.

If the shoulder is hurting, place the arm on the ribs. We are turning the rib cage and NOT attempting to dislocate the shoulder joint. Some people will be using the body to OVER MOVE the shoulder and arm for a "stiff" and "tight" mid-back. Essentially the person is slightly dislocating the shoulder which is causing the pain.

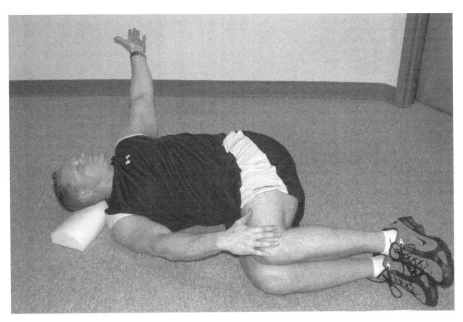

(Upper Spinal Twist)

CHAPTER THIRTEEN

Neck Pain

One patient came to my office recently complaining of left-wrist pain. I checked her upper kinetic chain by moving her shoulder blades together and nothing happened. I had her do Warrior 1 stretch from Yoga, to stretch the psoas and her wrist pain disappeared instantly.

This was not an isolated incident. A nice young couple brought their daughter in to see me. She had initially seen an orthopedist who had diagnosed her with *Dequervain's tenosynovitis,* a wrist tendon problem. The orthopedist recommended injections and if that failed, then surgery. Just like the patient above I had this 12 year old girl do a simple yoga stretch to affect the hip flexor and her pain went away instantly. Her mom, a psychologist, and father; an engineer, could not believe what happened. In less than 2 minutes the pain was gone.

What is the goal?: Treatment that is myopic or a Miracle? Wealthy people do not work like poor people. The BIG PICTURE is always in their mental framework. Pareto's law is the "guide" or goal, which is the 20% effort with the 80% result. Work smart, and not hard. We are "open" to anything and assume nothing.

I am NOT saying injections do not work or surgery is not on the table for some people but, if we can do a little stretch on a hip and the pain goes away in less than two minutes then why not?

It is sometimes difficult to explain to the patient how or why a seemingly unconnected part of the body is the cause of pain. I usually make the patient aware that she is not a neck, or a wrist, and that the body is a system or a unit. The neck or wrist is just one part of the body and we always need to think from a total body perspective. Alternatively, you could use the example of a car, which is not just an engine or tires, but a number of parts that work together to make the car what it is.

Neck-pain, arm numbness, and many shoulder pains are the result of the same problem. Pain in the traps is from the rectus femoris, or quads. I would also do some stretching of the psoas because I have seen that stretch relieve just about every complaint of pain. First, we need to find out if the pain is coming from the shoulder blades or if it is coming from the low-back. I tend to start with the low-back first because the majority of people have low-back problems even though the person does not complain.

Always do the MEB 3 protocol unless it breaks one of the commandments because this pattern resolves most patients' complaints. If the patient still has pain then try these:

1. **Quad stretch or kick in the butts** for pain in the traps, (the muscles that make body builders look like they have huge necks): stretch the quad with a quad stretch or kick in the butts.

154

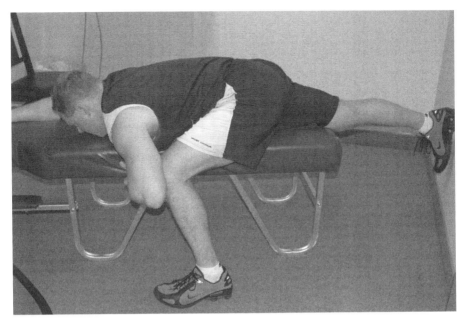

(Kick in the butts)

2. **Calf stretch**. Find a step stool or use a staircase. Place the feet on the edge of the step and then let the body weight drop down into the heels. Did the neck pain go away? Ok... keep doing it. 20% effort and 80% return. Do what works and nothing more and then leave it alone. The exercise can be repeated throughout the day. The mini stretching-breaks work best.

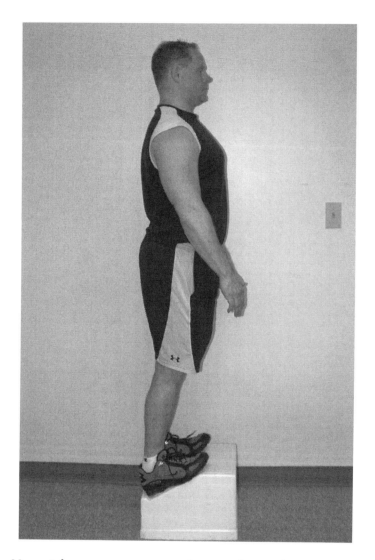

3. **Hamstrings**: use runner's stretch or the Shaolin stretch mentioned in Chapter Twelve.

4. **Frogs**. For pain in the side of the neck or scalene area, stretch the adductor magnus with supine PNF or prone frogs. Do not forget to ask the question on each stretch… "In this position how is your pain now?"

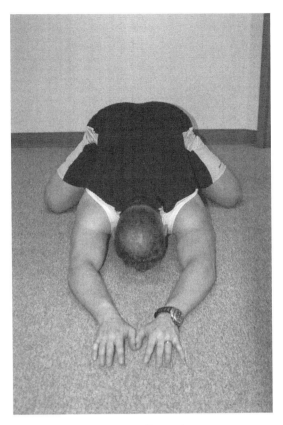

Prone Frogs)

5. **Seated glute meds, with band**. Sit in a chair and place a "mini-band" slightly above the knees. Now press the legs outward. Is this exercise helping? Is it 50% relief? If so then do it. If not, then DUMP it. If you have has a desk-job take the band to work with you and repeat the exercise periodically throughout the day. If you cannot find a "mini-band" at the local sports store or online, you cab use your hands and place them outside the knees. Press the legs into the hands while the hands are resisting. Did it help? Then do it.

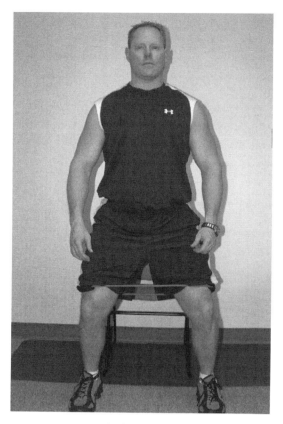

(Seated glut band meds)

6. **Pigeon-Toed Thigh Squeeze**. While the patient is standing, have her turn her toes in, or pigeon-toed. Now have the patient squeeze the thighs and straighten the legs. Hold that for a little bit and ask if the pain is going away. If the patient is feeling better, continue with the exercise. If not, stop. If this made it "worse" than do the opposite. Be open to anything and assume nothing. 20% effort and 80% result. Find that!

7. **Standing, Toes-Out-45-Degree-Angle, Glute Squeeze**. In the standing position, have the patient turn the toes out, and then squeeze the buttocks tightly. Squeeze and release for

about 10 reps and ask if the exercise is helping. If the pain level is improving, continue. If not, stop.

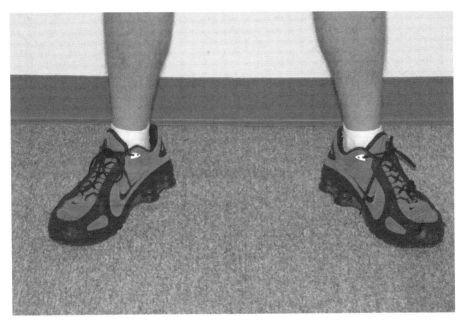

(Toes-out butt squeezes)

8. **Shoulder Blade Squeeze**. If none of the above-mentioned exercises are effective, check the position of the shoulder blades. Have the patient squeeze the shoulder blades together and see if the pain decreases. If the pain decreases, have the patient squeeze and release the shoulder blades 20 to 30 times.

9. **Tricep Kickbacks**. This exercise helps to synchronize the normal rhythmic movement of the arm with the leg while running or walking. Arm swing/leg swing. The arms need to be in harmony with the legs. When we run, our arms swing and pump up and down. The faster we pump the arms, the

faster the legs move. Many people who have neck pain actually have a shoulder problem/scapular problem.

Grab a light dumbbell or soup can, or some light-weighted object. Place the leg opposite the arm holding the "weighted" object forward, or step forward. Now bend over at the waist. Bring the elbow back to 90 degrees or parallel with the floor and then extend the elbow or take the weighted object towards the ceiling kicking the arm backwards; i.e., a "tricep kickback".

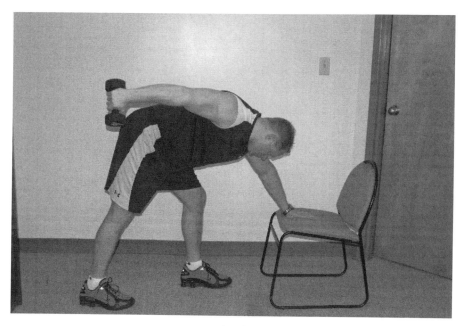

(Tricep kickbacks)

10. Lat Swings. This exercise can also be used for low-back pain. Have the patient stand in a runner's position and grab a dumbbell anywhere from 1 to 10 pounds. I start most patients with a three-pound dumbbell. Let the arm on the leg that is back hang down, while holding the dumbbell. Now swing the arm while keeping it straight up towards the ceiling and follow the movement with the head and eyes. We are using the powerful lat to pull the shoulder back into position. This is a great exercise to try when you are not sure what to do.

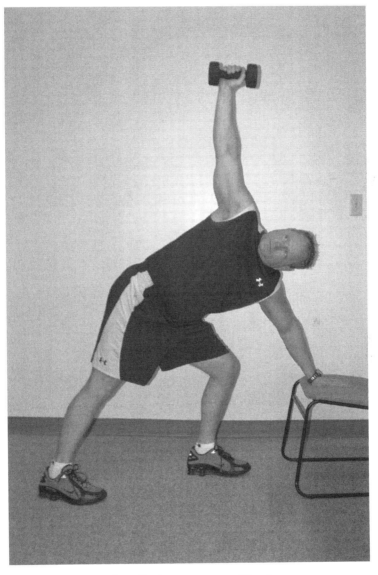

(Lat Swing, top position)

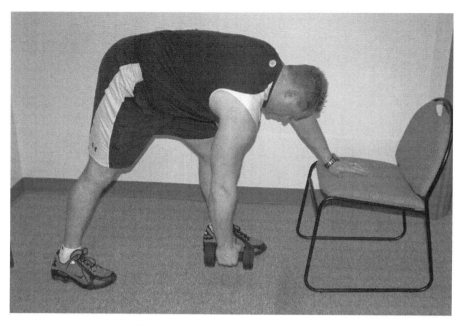

(Lat Swing, bottom position)

11. Standing or Seated Band Lat Row. Hook a band around a door hinge or around the therapist, pole or sturdy object. Have the patient squeeze the shoulder blades together and row the arms back. This exercise uses the strong and powerful lats and rhomboids to pull the shoulder blade back into position.

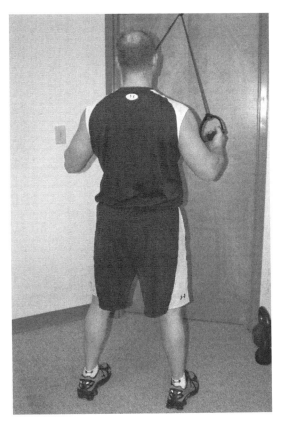

(Standing lat band row)

12. **Quadruped Position**. Have the patient get on all fours like a dog, or quadruped. Move the hips forward so that they are not directly above the knees and allow a natural curve to come into the low-back and the shoulder blades to come together. Remember to ask the patient, "In this position how is your neck pain now?" Also remember... **20% effort and 80% return. If any exercise is NOT helping, or helping very little, DUMP IT!**

163

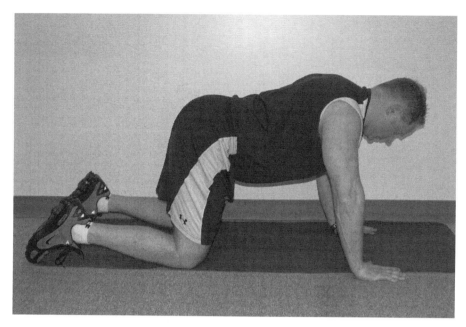

(Quadruped)

13. **Downward-Facing Dog**.   Have the patient get on all fours, quadruped. Now straighten the legs and walk the legs closer to the hands. The patient needs to be able to straighten the legs and then drop the heels. Now squeeze or tighten the thighs and push the tailbone towards the ceiling and back. This is a big stretch for most people, so be sure to ask the question, "In this position how is your neck pain now?" Make sure the patient lets the head hang down instead of trying to lift it. Lifting the head will increase neck pain, while letting it hang relaxed will relieve neck pain very quickly for many people.

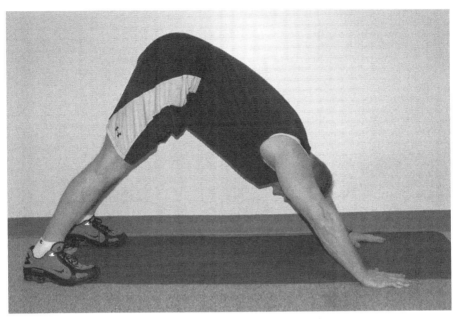

(Downward dog)

CHAPTER FOURTEEN

SINUS/COUGH

Many people have a sinus problem. They will attribute their sinus problem to the weather or an allergy, or provide some other reason for it. Frequently, the problem becomes a lifelong illness from which they get little relief. Some people have surgery to alleviate their sinus problem, only to have it return. This makes me think we are treating the symptom or affect as opposed to *the cause*.

I am not saying the surgeon is doing anything wrong; however, if we can make a change that does not require surgery, and the person begins to get well naturally; then, to me, that seems like a better option.

As far as allergies go some people may have an *anchor* that triggers the allergy. An anchor is a term used in *neurolinguistic programming* (NLP) that describes how a smell, feeling, or program is running behind the scenes. Take for example a song that comes on the radio and reminds us of a date, a moment, or place in our past. The same feelings and memories come back every time we hear that song. This is an anchor. The mind is very powerful. It can work for us, or it can work against us. Some patients may need to see an NLP therapist to correct the allergy. Other patients who have allergies and sinus problems respond well to medicine. Still others have responded very well to chiropractic treatment because their sinus problem or allergy is due to a mechanical or neurological problem.

If the patient has forward head posture (FHP), the neck muscles will tighten up. Forward head posture is when the head or "ear hole" is in front of the shoulders. For every inch the head moves forward the head increases in weight or the amount of stress on the neck.

If the neck muscles tighten up, they pull on the skull and could block lymph drainage, which is located in close proximity to the neck muscles. The tightened muscles could act like a dam to prevent the normal flow of lymph fluid, thus backing it up into the sinus cavity.

The body needs to move fluids around because this is the natural order of things. The ocean has currents, waves, and tides to churn the water. A river flows, and so does our blood. Our body is full of fluids that need to move; when one way is blocked, the fluid finds another route. If the body cannot move the lymph fluid one way, the body could discharge it through the nose or let it drip down the throat to the lung to be coughed up as phlegm. Our body is not out to harm us, but it does what it has to do to keep the system functioning.

Here are some stretches and exercises that will help relieve a sinus problem in a patient with FHP:

1. **Rectus Femoris/Quad Stretch**. This is the same stretch we used for neck pain and low-back pain, but now we employ it for sinus problems. If the rectus becomes too tight, it pulls the pelvis forward. As the pelvis moves forward, the head moves forward. Release the rectus, and the sinus on the

side you are stretching will open up. This also works for a cough. Try it and see. Many patients stop coughing after doing this stretch.

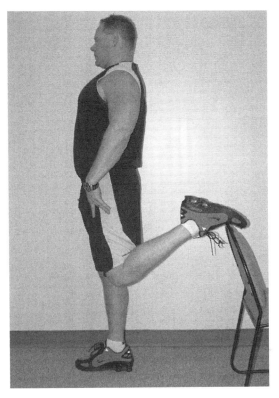

(Quad Stretch)

This stretch can be done standing, but it also can be done while lying on one's side or in a lunge position with half the body on the table. (I call this position, *kick in the butts*.) The person places one leg out in front of them on the floor like a lunge and the other leg is positioned on the table with the knee hanging off. Next, have the patient kick himself in the butt with his heel. Do five to seven reps and then PNF the quad.

169

To PNF the quad, grab the toes of the leg that is on the table and slowly and gently move the toes closer to the buttocks. Now, have the patient press the foot into your hand to lengthen out the muscle and create a new range of motion. Have the patient do this for about ten–fifteen seconds and relax. In the relax phase, bring the foot closer to the buttocks in a tolerable range. Do not hurt the patient, but do stretch him. Be careful because most patients' quads are very tight. When doing this, hold down the sacrum so that the patient cannot use the hip flexors and pelvic rotation to compensate. We are looking to lengthen the rectus and the rest of the hip flexors. I know it hurts; but the reward is well worth it.

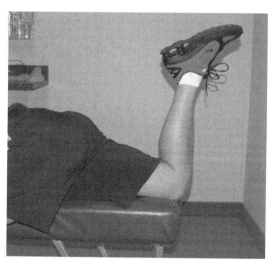

(Kick in the butts)

2. **Downward dog**. This releases dural tension and the sub occipital area will loosen up, relieving C1-C3, which is the area that supplies the nerves to the sinus and head. To understand why we are stretching the calves and hamstrings in this position, it is helpful to use a metaphor. Consider

this: if I pull on the bottom of your shirt where do you feel it? You feel it at the top. Using this idea, explain to the patient that the calves and hamstrings are pulling at the bottom, and they are just experiencing the pull at the top. I let go of the shirt and the tension releases.

Do not forget to ask the patient if the position is making him feel better or worse. If the patient feels better, stay with it. **20% effort... 80% returns**.

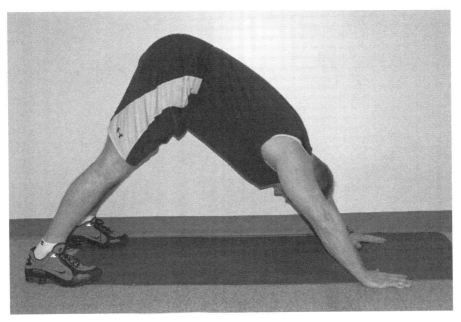

(Downward dog)

CHAPTER FIFTEEN

KNEE PAIN

Knee pain can be felt in the front, sides, or back of the joint, or in a combination of all these areas. Choosing the best course of treatment and then alleviating the pain depends upon where the pain is located. Most of the time, the underlying cause is a hip problem and pelvic instability. There also could be weakness of the medial hamstring; re-educating the medial hamstring effectively alleviates knee pain in many patients. Several remedies are listed in the following pages. It is not necessary to do every stretch or exercise listed in any protocol, but only those that alleviate the patient's pain.

1. **Quad Stretch**. Frontal pain (pain in the front of the knee) is usually due to the quad being too tight. Have the patient put his leg up behind him on a counter or bench. He should feel a stretch in the front of the quad. If the patient does not feel the stretch, or if he is very unstable, do kick in the butts instead.

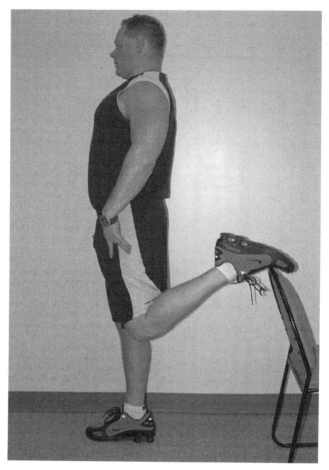

(Quad stretch)

2. **Runner's Stretch**. If the patient complains of lateral/posterior pain (back or side of leg), have him face a table or chair, and stride out a little into a forward lunge. The legs should be lined up with the hips. Now, the patient should bend at the waist and squeeze the quad on the leg that is forward while resting his arms on the table for balance. If the person is okay, then have him move away from the bench or chair and go down as far as he can. Again, squeeze the forward leg's quad or thigh muscles.

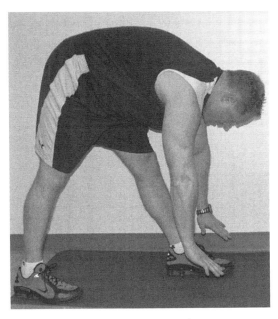

(Runner's Stretch)

3. **Prone Cox Leg Circles for Anterior Femoral Glide**. Many knee pains, and pains in general, are due to anterior femoral glide. When a patient walks, the leg that is moving backward at the beginning of the movement is starting with the hamstring instead of the glutes and the deep glute stabilizers. So the hipbone has moved forward, causing the knee to become unstable. The hamstring becomes overworked and now it complains.

   To alleviate this problem, have the patient lie on a table or exercise ball on his stomach. Make sure the back is in a neutral position and there is no pressure on it. Now goad (dig) the glute with the knuckles of your fist, being careful not to exert too much pressure. This gets the glute muscles to begin firing. Next, have the patient raise his leg. If the hamstring fires first, stop the leg raise. If the patient arches or recruits the low-back as evidenced by an increased curve or SI joint motion, stop the stretch or have the patient lower his leg a little bit.

175

If the patient is having a hard time getting the glute to fire, then have the person take the arm on the same side and grab the table. This will open up the L5 area of the low-back and get the lat to fire, thereby stabilizing the SI joints.

After the patient raises his leg with the foot straight, paying close attention to details listed above, have him turn the foot to the outside at the hip socket and raise the leg. Next, have the patient turn the foot to the inside and raise the leg. Make sure the glute is firing before raising the leg. Turning the foot in also builds up the medial hamstring. This alleviates most knee pain rather quickly and improves total body position.

I must also make you aware that this stimulates quite a bit of parasympathetic input and the patient can feel a little woozy after doing this. Secondly, the patient's center of gravity will change, so he frequently feels different after doing this exercise.

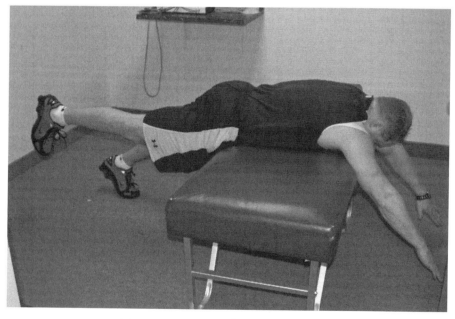

(Anterior Femoral Glide Patterns)

4. **Standing with Foot Turned In**. I like the anterior femoral glide work the best, but if a patient is in a hurry, do this one. In addition, this one is a standing exercise so we have a lot more neurological integration than when the patient is lying down. Get close to a wall for support. Now, turn the foot in and then lift the leg backward. Many knee pains will be gone in seconds with this exercise.

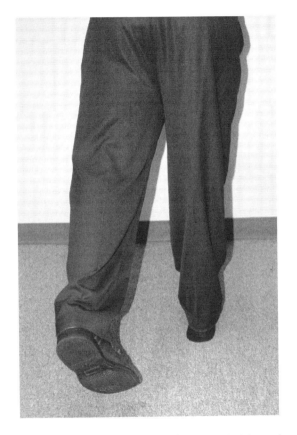

5. **Seated glute med bands**. Take a mini-band and place it around both ankles, then bring it to a level right above the knees. Have the patient sit down and spread the legs apart so that tension is on the band. Next, have the patient push the band out to the side. You can do this for reps or you

can have the patient hold it there. Do not forget to ask the patient questions as he is doing the exercise or stretch. Push out. Ask him how it feels. If he senses improvement, continue the exercise.

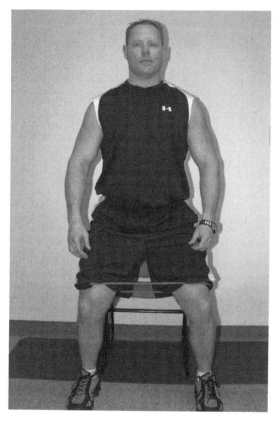

(Seated glut band meds)

6. **Calf stretch**. A great overall stretch for just about any condition from headaches to low-back and of course, knee pain. Have the patient stand on a slant board, SOT blocks, or a step where his calves can drop down to stretch. Stay on the slant until the calves feel even and loose. Some people may be so tight that they fall backward. Position the patient close

to a wall for support or hold on to a stair railing. Again, ask if the stretch is making the patient feel better.

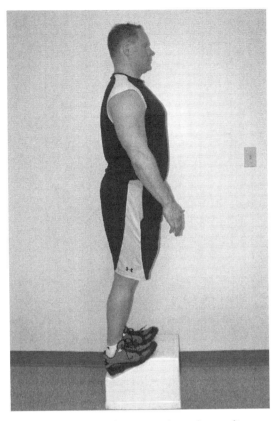

(Calf stretch on a slant board)

7. **Janda Sit-Ups**. The patient needs to lie on his back and place his legs over a table or exercise ball, pushing the heels into the ball or table. Then the patient must try to sit up. This activates the hamstrings and inhibits/prevents the hip flexor from engaging. The patient is isolating the abs to create core stability. Many knee pains and most other pains originate from a lack of hip and core stability.

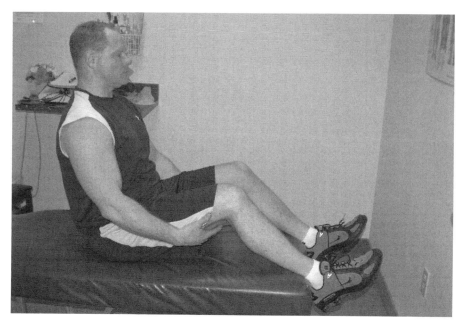

(Janda Sit-ups)

CHAPTER SIXTEEN

HIP PAIN

The hips generate power. They are the impetus for most of our movements and are connected to the strongest kinetic (movement) chain in our body. The hips are close to the body's center of gravity, which is located at S2-S3.

There is a Bible story about a man named Jacob, who wrestled with God. According to the story, God touched Jacob on the hip socket and, as a result, Jacob walked with a limp for the rest of his life. Babies are made through hip motion. The hip is an amazing joint when it works the way it is designed to work. If we get these powerful joints working correctly, moving through the day becomes very easy.

Very few people complain of hip pain, but they will complain of IT band pain or a locking or "popping out" sensation in the hip socket. For a time I was baffled by IT band pain. Stretching the IT band resulted in very little relief for the patient. Then I remembered my own philosophy that it might be somewhere else! There are a few stretches in close proximity to the hip that can help, but the relief comes when we work well above the hip. I am going to give you two ways to address the problem. One is to go into the problem to some degree, and the other is to leave it alone.

Scenario number one: going into it...

1. **Kick in the butts.** This exercise has been explained previously, so I'll save some time and paper and ask you to please refer to the photograph below. You can do this one, or the quad stretch. I prefer kick in the butts because it adds mobility, which is an improved functional range of motion. However, standing quad stretch adds the component of balance, which is also very important. One or the other will help with IT band pain and hip pain.

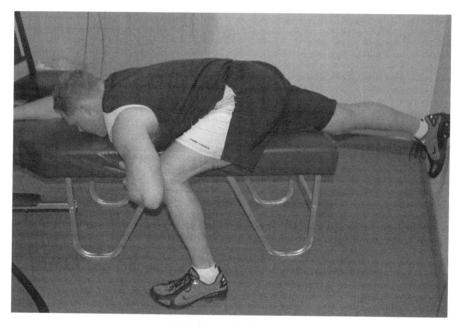

(Kick in the butts)

2. **Kneeling Warrior 1**. Kneel in a half kneeling position. Squeeze the glutes and do NOT feel any "pinching" or "pain" in the low-back. Now move forward and allow the thigh muscles to release. One can kneel on a gardener pad that can be purchased at *Home Depot* or some other garden store. Or one can place a pillow under the knee.

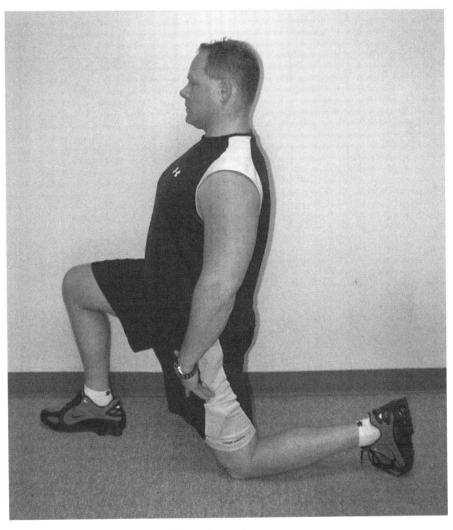

(Kneeling Warrior)

183

3. **Calf Stretch**. Have the patient stand on a slant board, on SOT blocks, or a step where the patient's calves can drop down to stretch. Stay on the slant until the calves feel even and loose. Some patients may be so tight that they fall backward. Move the patient close to a wall for support. Again, is it making the patient better?

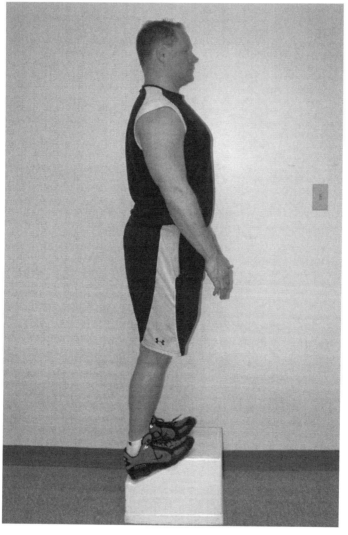

(Calf stretch)

4. **Add Mag/Frogs**. Get on all fours. Now spread the legs apart. Some people might need some padding or cushions for the knees. Again, we could use some foam pads that gardeners use, or pillows. Relax and breathe. Don't force the stretch. One should feel it in the inner thighs or "groin area".

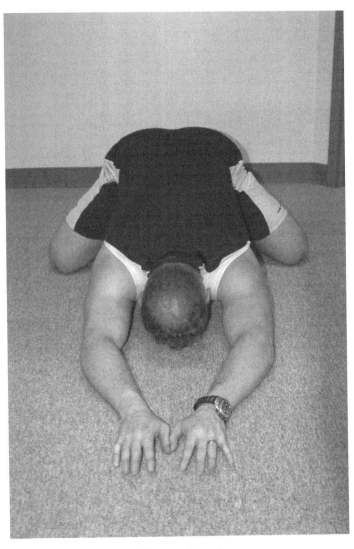

(Prone Frog)

5. **Standing Table Top or "L"**. Feet are hip width apart. Use a chair, a counter top or wall and then bend over at the waist so that the body forms an "L", or 90 degree angle. Keep the legs straight and "lock" the knees. The upper body is to relax and so should the stomach muscles.

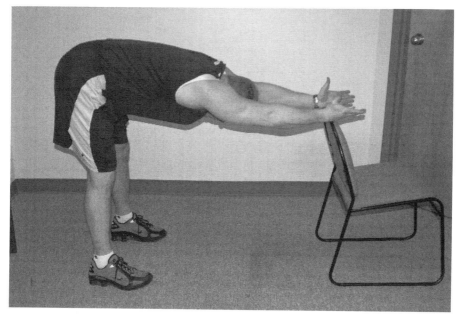

(Table top or "L")

6. **Anterior Femoral Glide** as shown below:

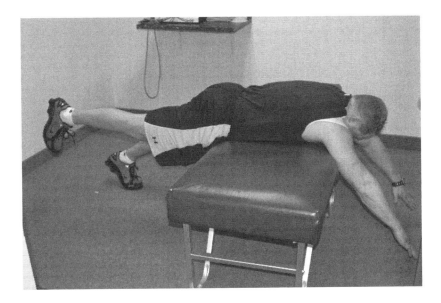

7. **Superman Table/Sorensen's test**

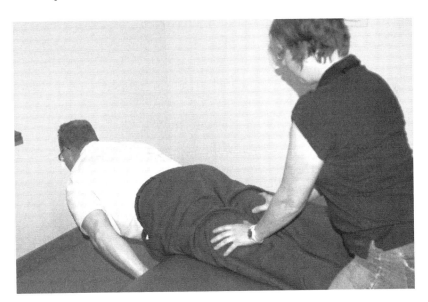

8. **Spiderman**. Have the patient step out into a 2 o'clock lunge. The forward leg should be at 90 degrees, at the knee and the right arm is gliding down the inside of the leg to touch the floor. The other arm can go to the floor as well for support. This will open up the hip sockets and create a huge global stretch of the hips, legs, and back. After 2 o'clock is held for at least 30 seconds—and up to 2 minutes—then go to the 10 o'clock position. Now let the left arm slide down the inside of the left leg. The front leg should be at 90 degrees, and the back leg should be straight.

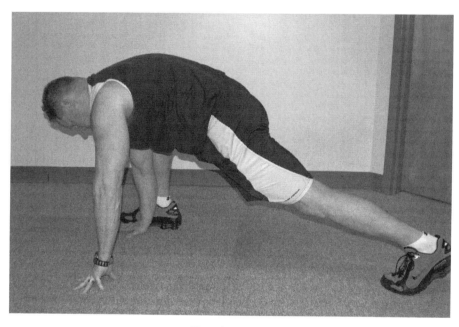

(Spiderman)

188

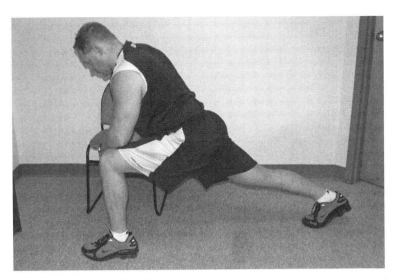

(Modified Spiderman with a chair)

9. **Band Squats High to Low**. This exercise is great for elderly people and middle-agers who are really stiff. Put a mini-band on and bring it up to right above the knees. Do this while the patient is sitting. Now have the patient stand up with the mini-band on and make sure the patient pushes the knees out when sitting and standing. Have the patient do five reps and, of course, ask the question, "How is the pain now?"

I usually have the patient do about ten reps, then I progress the person to a lower chair or bench, and then to a 12-inch stool. The patient may need help getting up, but keep working at it. The knees must push out as the patients sits, and then stands. Remember: Knees out.

If the patient has a severe balance problem, do not progress him to the 12-inch stool. Also make sure the stool is next to a wall so that if the patient begins to lose his balance he can use the wall for support. It is understood, but I will say it for emphasis: spot the patient. Hold his hands until the body catches on. The goal here is function, pain relief, and safety.

A third way of doing the band squat is to use a doorframe. Simply have a patient face the doorframe and hold the frame as he slowly squats down. Make sure the back is straight and upright.

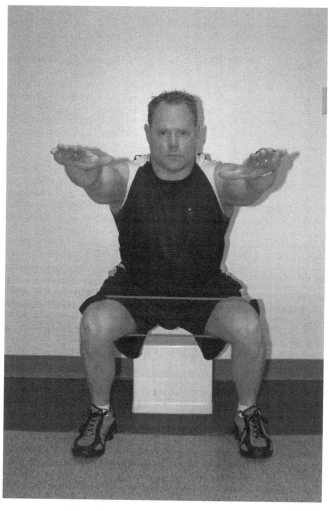

(Band squat on 12 inch stool)

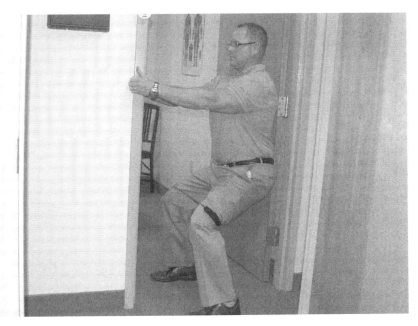

(Doorway band squat)

10. Sumo Squat Walks. This exercise can also be used for low-back pain. A word of caution: this exercise is to be used only if the patient has a good sense of balance. Patients who are unsteady on their feet, elderly, or have had a knee or hip replacement, are not candidates for this exercise.

Have the patient stand with his feet turned out at a 45-degree angle and the legs placed wider than hip width. The patient will then squat down like a Sumo wrestler. Next, the patient is going to squat and walk at the same time. The knees need to push out hard. This is a really effective exercise for the quads and glutes. Additionally, the patient will have a greater range of hip motion and less pain. If you are unsure or scared then do not do this exercise. This is an aggressive move so try it yourself first, master it, and then use it carefully with a patient. Don't forget the rule... 20% effort and

191

80% return. Do a little bit to see if it helps and make sure that the exercise is NOT irritating or increasing the pain. Please check with the patient first before doing a series of Sumo squat walks. This is a dynamic mobility exercise for the hips.

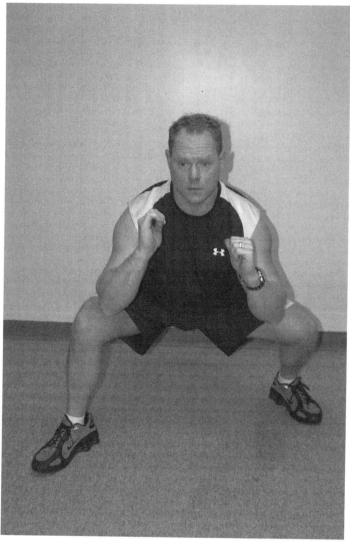

(Sumo squat walks)

11. **Curtseys**. This exercise is also on the aggressive side. Adhere to this rule of thumb: if you do not think the patient can do it safely, *do not do it*! In the standing position, have the patient step a leg behind the other leg like doing a *curtsey*. This is a mobility-move that will stretch the IT band while at the same time creating some hip stability on the opposite side.

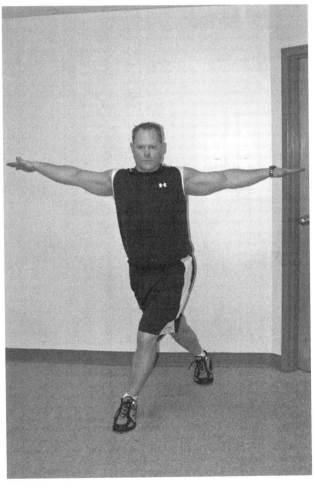

(Curtseys)

12. **Shaolin Leg Raise Up and Out to the Side**. Stand on one leg and raise the other leg up, bringing the knee toward the chest. Now, externally rotate the raised leg until it is parallel to the floor and hold. This requires a great deal of stability from the opposite hip and core. This exercise moves into functional exercises and mobility patterns. If the patient cannot do it without support, have him stand at arm's-length away from a wall. Now, raise the inside leg (leg closest to the wall) towards the shoulder and then out toward the wall.

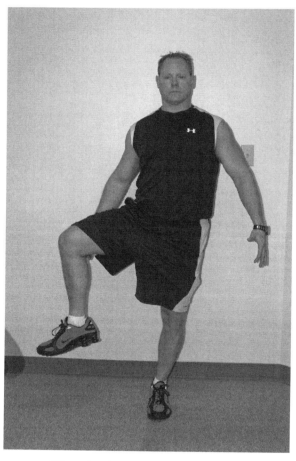

(Shaolin leg raise, out to side)

13. Lat Rows. Strengthening the *latissimus dorsi* helps to fix the shoulders and upper body to the hips/pelvis.

The *latissimus dorsi* acts like the IT band of the upper extremity, stabilizing the sacroiliac joints and synchronizing arm/leg swing as seen in walking. If the hip or low-back is irritated, the lat might not be working as it should and the IT band is becoming overloaded. **Remember, the part that is complaining is doing all of the work.** I have seen remarkable improvement in many of my patients when I move away from the IT band and the hip. I have seen patients with shin splints and foot pains on the outside of the ankle get better instantly. One of my patients is a collegiate gymnast who complained of severe shin splints; the lat row exercise relieved her pain instantly.

She asked me, "How does this happen?" I told her about the triangles of the upper body and lower body. Again the hardest thing in all of this is not the actual method, but explaining to a patient how, and why it works.

Remember Pareto's Law: 20% effort and 80% return. Does one want to work 12 hour days for $300/week or does one want to work 2 hours/day for $100,000/week?

If one hops on the right leg all day long is it possible the right leg will hurt? Is the right leg the issue or is it that the person might want to get the "left leg" to help out? In this case... we are asking the lats to help out. We are OPEN to anything vs. just a quick snap judgment, and myopic or "narrow view" of the issue.

To do this exercise you will need a long band that has handles on it. Place the band on the top hinge of a door. (Some band kits come with a strap that allows you to slide it over the band and then close the door to fix the band at whatever height you desire.) In this case, I want the band at the top of the door.

Now, have the patient grab the handles with palms up. Have the patient squeeze his glutes, which will stabilize and protect the hips and low-back. We do not want to engage the upper body if the lower body is unstable. Next, have the patient extend the arms to straighten them out and pull both arms back. This will engage the triceps and lats at the same time pulling the shoulders back into position. In this position ask the question, "How is the pain now?" Most patients will tell you that the pain is gone.

There are two ways of doing this, reps or a static hold; both are effective.

Static holds means just pull the band back and "hold it" there. *Reps,* or repetitions, means down and up or back and forth. I like the static hold best because the longer the person holds it, the greater the nervous system fires with tension on it. I recommend standing behind the patient to help him bring his shoulders back and his chest up. This exercise is done while the patient is in a normal postural alignment.

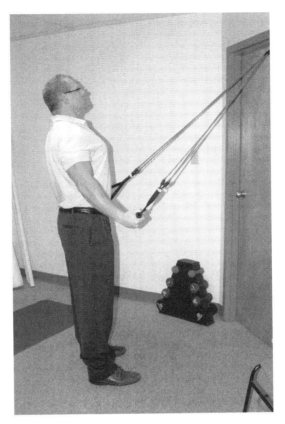

(Lat rows)

If you do not have bands, use a dumbbell and do lat swings. Have the patient step into a lunge position while using a bench or chair for support. Hold a dumbbell (no heavier than 10 lbs.) in the hand on the open leg side. Example: left leg back, dumbbell in left hand. In the lunge position, right hand on the chair for support, have the patient raise her left arm toward the ceiling while keeping it straight. This will open up the torso and engage the lat. This exercise also relieves shoulder pain and low-back pain. Do five reps and ask the patient about her level of pain. If the pain is reduced, work up to 10 reps. Do the exercise on the other side as long as the patient is not complaining of pain.

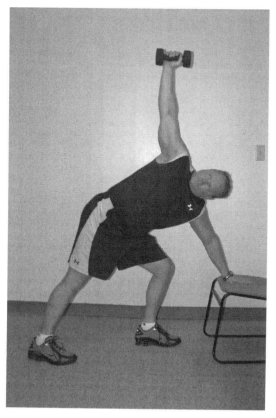

(Lat swings)

14. **Wide-Stance Air Chair**. This exercise is not only good for hip pain, but also low-back, neck, arm radiculopathy (pain down the arm) and shoulder pain. Use this exercise to figure out what has the body off balance and restore the hips as the body's center of gravity. This is why it works. We are putting the body back in alignment with its center of gravity.

Ask the patient to stand against a door and then walk her feet out with the legs spread out wider than shoulder width.

Next, ask the patient to squat down while pushing the knees out hard. The patient's tailbone should be against the door as she continues to slide down as far as possible.

Some patients will feel as if they are going to fall. Stay close for support, but encourage them to descend as far as possible, getting the hips below the knees if possible. I learned this exercise from a patient who is an avid skier. I tried it on my hip problem and achieved immediate relief. Do not forget to ask the question, "In this position how is your pain now?" If better, continue. If worse, stop; but only if the patient is complaining about joint pain. Do not stop because a patient feels a muscle burn.

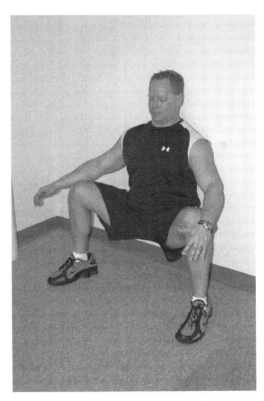

(Wide stance air chair or wall squat)

Scenario number two: leave it alone…

Scenario number two is to leave the hip problem alone. There is an acupuncture theory that teaches not to add stimulation to an area that is already super stimulated. The first scenario works the hip joint with exercises in and around the hip. The second scenario does not involve any hip joint exercises; instead, the exercises focuses on the upper body and torso.

The body can be divided into two triangles placed on top of each other. The lower triangle is comprised of the pelvis and legs. The upper triangle is comprised of the lats to the upper body.

It is my theory that when the lower triangle is over stimulated, the problem will likely be found in the upper triangle. The protocol above may work, and it may not. If the protocol above is not effective, we need to find another method.

Always remember the premise of the book, which is to do what works and do not create more pain. Remember that I am NOT in the room with the patient, so I cannot see the way the patient moves or hear him describe his pain. Therefore, what I offer is a guide, or set of tools, that typically work with a high degree of effectiveness.

If the above method is not effective, the protocol described below may be helpful.

Also remember to keep it simple. Keep your thought process simplistic. Sometimes muscles want to be stretched and sometimes they do not. Sometimes muscles need to be strengthened and sometimes strengthening makes it worse. Sometimes we will do exercises for the front of the body and they are effective, and sometimes it makes it worse. If working on one side of the body makes things worse, then try the other side of the body; e.g., front made worse, then start working the back muscles. If working on the front and back make the patient feel worse, try something on the side like the muscles on the left and right sides of the body. If front-to-back and side-to-side does not work, try turning motions or turning stretches. If I am working on the bottom half of the body, and the patient is feeling worse, maybe I need to work the top half.

Keep thinking about balance. Life is a simple balance equation; too much of this and not enough of that. What do we need to do to bring about balance? Review the simplistic thought processes I just presented in the preceding paragraph. Try the front and I have two choices... stretch or strengthen? If both say "no," then move to the next area.

If I tried working on the front and nothing was effective, I think about strengthening the back. Or maybe it is stretch the front and strengthen the back? Or vice versa? I keep looking for the combination of exercises and stretches that work, or even the one thing that is effective. The body/brain will lead the way. We are using the most technical and sophisticated piece of equipment ever developed: the human brain. Marvel at that and not the MRI. The brain can guide the doctor and patient to the answer. The MRI can only show me a picture. It offers no real guidance that what we propose to do will be effective. On the other hand, the brain can give me instantaneous, real-time feedback, and the MRI cannot.

Again, determine which of the tools I have provided works best for the patient. When you get it right, the patient will quickly become pain free. Sometimes it takes a series of exercises and stretches to alleviate a hip problem because it is such an integral part of the system.

1. **Janda Sit-Ups**. The body's core/abdomen needs to engage to control the movement required for a patient to squat or sit down. If the upper body and torso become unstable, other areas make up for the instability, usually the IT band and hip sockets. Janda sit-ups will create the core stability needed for squatting or going from a standing position to sitting.

   Janda sit-ups are not like the sit-ups most people are familiar with from gym class. Dr. Janda, a world-renowned bio mechanist and neurologist, uses reciprocal inhibition to override the overactive and dominant hip flexor. Most people have turned their hip flexor into a "trunk flexor." The mechanics of a typical sit-up require the person to use the hip flexor to make up for a weak abdomen, which causes low-back pain, and many a disc bulge and/or herniation. This result is what makes people believe that sit-ups are bad exercises and should not be done. Janda sit-ups correct the bad mechanics of the typical sit up.

   As the abdomen becomes stronger and has the ability to stabilize the core/spine, the hip flexor can go back to being a hip flexor. Balance returns to the system, and hip pain disappears.

   Person: "I heard sit-ups are bad for you."

   Answer: An exercise is not a "good" or "bad" thing. It is whether an exercise is causing a person a problem or not. For some people sit-ups are not helpful, but for others they could be beneficial.

There are several ways of using Janda's principle for the sit-up. One method is to use a chair or exercise ball and while the patient is lying on her back have her push the heels into the ball or chair. Next, have the person crunch up or attempt a sit-up.

Another method is to have the patient lie on her back on a table, scooting down so that the heels are off the table and the knees are slightly bent. Now have the patient sit up, or you can have the patient start in the sit-up position and then lean back as far as she can while controlling the movement. Then have the patient come back up to the original position again.

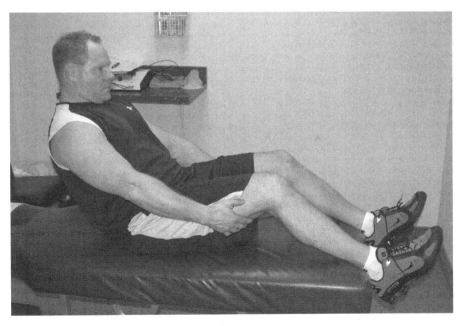

(Janda sit-up)

2. **Janda with Russian Twist**. Have the patient stay in the up position of the sit-up, and then slowly descend to a point

about halfway or less. Extend both arms and clasp hands together, palm-to-palm. Now take both arms and turn the upper body left and hold, and then right and hold. We are engaging the obliques; the internal oblique shares connections with the *transversus abdominous*. The obliques attach the pelvis to the rib cage and create the stability for power generated from the hips to the upper body. If the upper body becomes unstable, the body will become overloaded as a person stands, walks, and lifts. This exercise corrects the weakness and creates the needed stability, taking pressure or stress off of the IT bands and hip sockets.

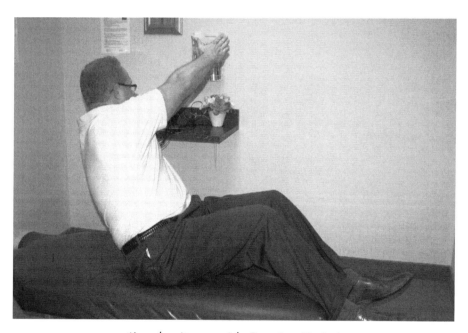

(Janda sit-up with Russian Twist)

3. **Reverse Hyperextensions**. Reverse hyperextensions require an exercise ball. I prefer a 55 cm ball because it is just the right height for patients who have poor balance and need to be closer to the ground, while at the same time offering

enough clearance to do the exercise. With the patient on his stomach over a 55 cm ball, have him go forward so that the hips are on the ball and the elbows are on the floor. The idea is to get the patient's upper body stable so that he can lift both legs up. The ball acts as a fulcrum of support; with the elbows on the ground we have good contact, which creates an easy leverage point to raise the legs.

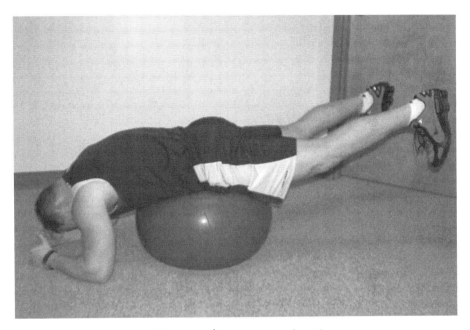

(Reverse hyperextensions)

4. **Upper Spinal Twist**. This exercise is more of a mobility exercise; it improves the body's range-of-motion by lengthening the obliques. When a muscle becomes shortened, it becomes weak. This exercise is from Yoga and we are using it here to alleviate IT band and hip pain and hip movement disorders created from core-instability issues.

205

Have the person lie on the floor on his side. Now bring both knees up to beltline level and bend the knees at a 90-degree angle. There will be a 90-degree angle where the leg and body meet, and a 90-degree angle at the knee to the foot. The position is similar to the fetal position. The neck should be comfortable. Some patients may need a pillow or some form of head support.

Now take the arm that is closest to the floor and place the hand on top of both knees. The knees need to be stacked in line and the hips/pelvis need to be in line. Now take the top arm and reach back for the floor. Do not force the movement, but allow the body to move only as far as it can. When the patient feels tension, have her relax into it and breathe several times. The breathing will relax the muscles allowing for a greater range. Forcing will engage the neurological reflexes and the body will push back against the patient, inhibiting motion.

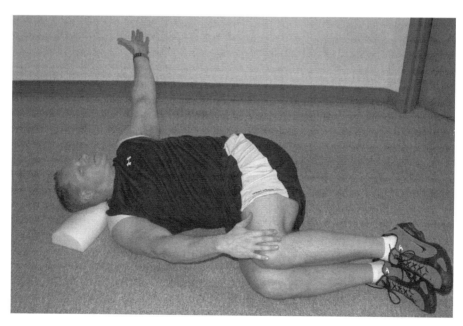

(Upper Spinal Twist)

5. **Foam Roll or Pillow Lower Spinal Twist**. Now that we have established some mobility in the upper part of the body, we are going to have the shoulders remain still and have the hips dissociate (move away) from the trunk. This motion occurs in all kinds of athletic activities and is part of everyday living.

Have the patient lie on his back and place a rolled-up towel under the head if needed. Bend both knees and bring them up toward the shoulders. Place a rolled-up towel, pillow, foam roll, or ball between the legs. Now place the arms out to the side, at a 90-degree angle. Now flip one hand palm-up and the other hand palm-down on the floor. Squeeze the shoulder blades together. Do not let the shoulder blades come apart or off of the floor. We are looking for stability and not whether the patient can take his legs to the side.

Have the patient *move the legs to the side of the palm-down hand* and then return to the center position. Do 3 to 10 reps to one side, then 3 to 10 reps to the other side. Make sure the back remains elongated, tall, when doing the exercise. Do not forget to reverse the hands when going to the other side and keep the shoulder blades squeezed and on the floor.

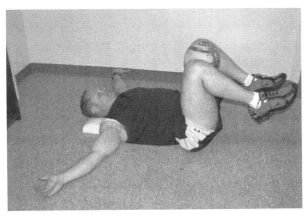

(Lower Spinal Twist or hip dissociation)

6. **Ball Seated Chop and Lift**. Sit on an exercise ball and hold another ball, weight, or clasp hands together out in front of the body. The arms should be straight. Now position the arms over one knee while sitting up tall on the ball. Next, raise the arms up and over the opposite shoulder. Most patients will not be able to go over the shoulder with the arms, but the idea is to create this chopping and lifting effect. This exercise will help engage the rotational muscles of the body. See Tom Myer's book, *Anatomy Trains*, to understand the principles of what appears to be a relief from pain, or a *miracle*, by affecting a distant part of the body.

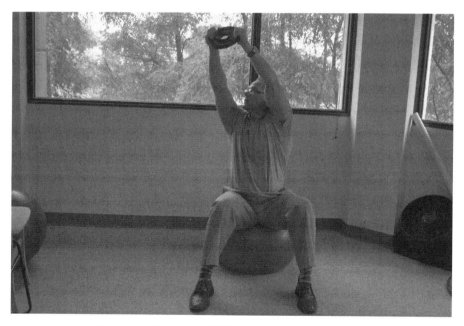

(Seated Chop and Lift on an exercise ball)

7. **Form Running**. Have the patient stand facing a wall; he needs to be about two feet away from the wall. Now have the patient place both hands on the wall like a wall pushup.

Tense all the muscles in the body, especially the glute, on the down leg because the other leg is going to come up towards the same side shoulder. Do 5–10 reps on one side, then do the other side; however, do not let the patient swing out too far to the side to do the exercise. Stand next to the down leg side, blocking the patient from listing to complete the exercise. The listing affect is part of what is creating the IT band pain, hip pain or low-back pain. The patient swings way out to the side to raise the opposite leg, which is very inefficient as far as walking and running goes. The person is working too hard to walk due to muscle imbalances.

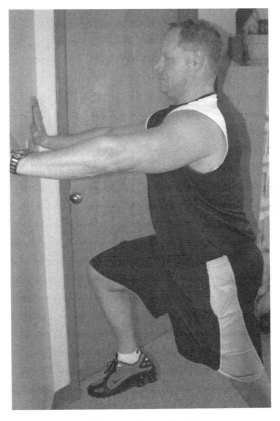

(Form Running)

CHAPTER SEVENTEEN

MID-BACK PAIN

Mid-back pain is often the result of the body recruiting the upper-back muscles to stabilize the lower back. Common methods of addressing the pain include stretching the area, rubbing it, massaging it, and then just giving it some time. Some patients' backs are so tight and stiff, that trying to do a chiropractic adjustment on the area is like pounding on a steel door.

I have taken the approach of using multi-joint positioning techniques to alleviate the pain, which has proven to be highly effective in alleviating most of my patients' pain. Again, this is not the cure, but if we can get patients some relief, then we can quickly reassure the patient that we can help them. The cure involves a series of steps to restore the patient's body to its optimum design.

Following is a list of exercises to use to relieve mid-back pain. You will need to experiment to see which exercises are effective in alleviating the symptom.

1. **Yoga Tabletop**. Have the patient face a counter or wall, placing his hands on the counter or wall. Next, have the patient walk his feet away from the counter or wall so that

211

the arms extend out, elbows straight and then bend over, forming an "L". Now, squeeze the quads to create flexion in the hips and push the buttocks back away from the counter or wall. The patient will feel a big stretch in the upper back, shoulders, and legs. This is a multi-jointed approach to the problem. Of course ask the question, "In this position how is the pain?" If the stretch is decreasing or improving the pain, or producing relief, then have the patient stay in the position until the pain is completely gone. If the stretch does not help, move on to another one. **We are NOT exercising or stretching for the sake of exercising.** We are doing activity that produces RESULTS or the desired goal... *as I continue to stress, the 20% effort and 80% result.*

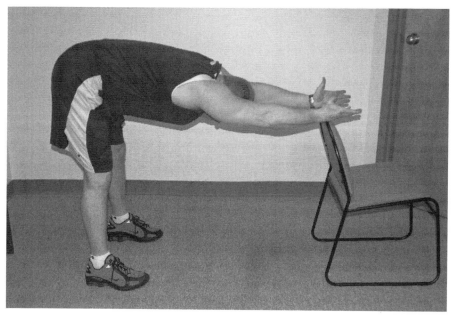

(Tabletop or "L")

2. **Prone pillow squeeze**. Have the patient lie on a table or floor, bending the knees so that the feet are parallel with the ceiling. Now place a pillow between the ankles and have the patient squeeze it. Squeeze and release repeatedly, or squeeze and hold. In the squeeze and hold position check to see what happened to the pain. Is it gone? If so, keep doing it. If not, move on to a different stretch.

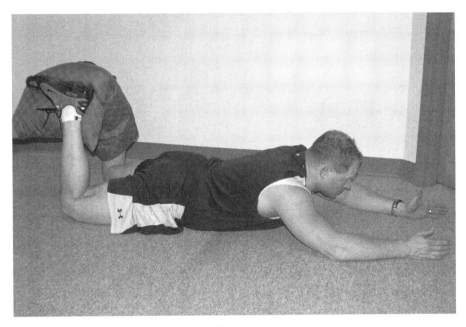

(Prone pillow squeezes)

3. **Quad Stretch or Kick in the Butts**. By now, you should realize that the quad stretch or *kick in the butts* resolve many a problem. A majority of patients have "quad dominance" and tight hip flexors, and since the lower part of the hip flexor attaches to the front of the pelvis, it pulls the pelvis anterior/forward. This creates an increase in thoracic kyphosis, or "hunchback" form, and a forward-head position.

To do kick in the butts, the patient places one leg out in front of him on the floor like a lunge, with the other leg positioned on the table with the knee hanging off. Next, have the patient kick himself in the butt with his heel. Do 5–7 reps and then PNF the quad by having the patient stop trying to strike the buttocks. Then grab the toes and slowly and gently move the toes closer to the buttocks. Now have the patient press the foot into your hand to lengthen out the muscle and create a new range of motion. Have the patient do this for about 10–15 seconds and relax. In the relax phase, bring the foot closer to the buttocks in a tolerable range. Do not hurt the patient, but do stretch him. Be careful because most people are very tight.

If you don't have a friend then get a rope, towel or even a little extension cord to wrap around the foot. Use the "rope" to pull the leg towards the buttocks and be gentle.

If you have a "buddy" they can hold the low-back down or even "sit" on the buttocks so that the person cannot use the hip flexors and pelvic rotation to compensate. We are looking to lengthen the rectus and the rest of the hip flexors. I know it hurts, but the reward is well worth it.

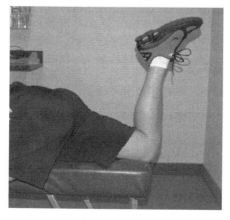

(Kick in the butts)

4. **Supine Psoas Strengthening**. With the patient on his back with legs bent and feet on the table. Now bring the knee up to the same side shoulder. Now apply pressure to the top of the knee for resistance. Hold this for about 10 seconds.

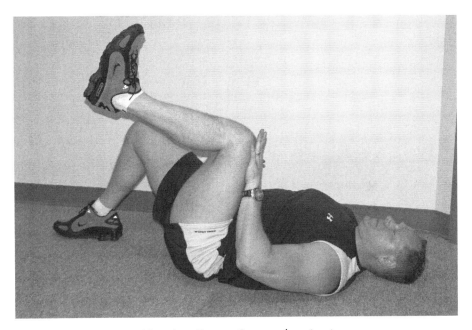

(Supine Psoas Strengthening)

5. **Quadruped**. Have the patient get on all fours like a dog, or quadruped. Now move the hips forward so that they are not directly above the knees, allowing a natural curve to come into the low-back and the shoulder blades to come together. Ask, "How is the pain in this position?" If the pain goes away or is going away then stay there. A person will know in 20-30 seconds. If it is helping then stay there. For example, the person has a 6/10 for mid-back pain and within 10 seconds ask, "What is the pain number now?" If the person goes a "4/10" then check again in 20 seconds and it is a "2/10" then... BAM... we found the 80/20 exercise. If

215

nothing is happening or it is increasing the pain then STOP. **This RULE applies to ALL the exercises in this book.** Our natural habit is to just do things without measuring RESULTS or PROGRESS.

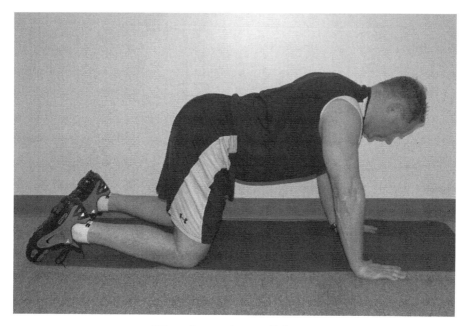

(Quadruped, or all fours)

CHAPTER EIGHTEEN

FOOT/ANKLE/SHIN PAIN

The foot is an integral body part. There is a theory that goes like this: Foot stable, ankle mobile, knee stable, hip stable and mobile, low-back stable, mid-back mobile and neck stable and mobile. It all begins with a stable foot.

We use the foot to stand. The ankle allows movement and transfers energy throughout the body. Most people today have problems with the "stable" foot. As people move, they are off balance and we can see that in how their shoes wear. Typically, the outside of the shoe wears out and often one side wears more than the other.

There are a variety of shoes that have been designed to support the foot and negate the natural movement of the body. We take apart, the foot, which has five individual segments, wrap it in leather and prevent it from properly moving. The five individual parts are now operating as one, which is not the way it is designed to work.

Athletes frequently tape their ankles or feet for support or to prevent injury. Ironically, taping prevents the part from moving the way it is designed to move. The ankle does not get stronger rather it gets weaker because the athlete relies on the tape for support instead of relying on his muscles. My theory is that we should return the body to its original design and specifications. We do that through corrective strategies rather than masking problems.

The foot is an area that many want to *mess around* with. In this book I am not offering cures, but ways to break pain patterns. What I offer in this chapter are effective protocols for alleviating foot, ankle, and shin pain.

1. **Lat rows**. I know this is surprising, but shin splints or pain on the outside of the calf will improve in minutes with lat rows. Get a band, put it on a door, and row away. Have the patient do about 10 reps with good posture. Chest up and open, butt squeezed (protecting the low-back) and legs straight.

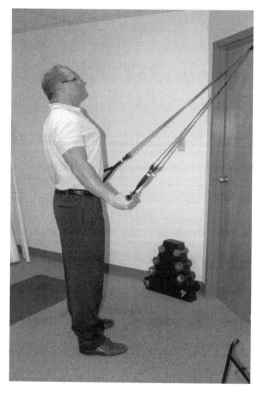

(Lat Rows)

2. **Psoas strengthening**. One of my patients was having such severe foot pain that he had scheduled surgery to try to correct the problem. I had him do the psoas-strengthening move and his pain was relieved by 90% in minutes. The reason is that the calf muscles are trying to perform the job of some of the hip muscles. The body is simply recruiting other muscles to stabilize the system or perform the action or both, which is what causes pain.

Have the patient lie on his back with both knees bent, bringing one knee up toward the same shoulder. Next, apply resistance to the top of the knee using an isometric contraction. Hold this for about 10 seconds and do not forget to ask, "How is the pain now?" If it is gone, keep doing the exercise. We also have an exercise that the patient can do to get relief any time he or she needs it. Adjusting the hip and ankle will also help alleviate this problem.

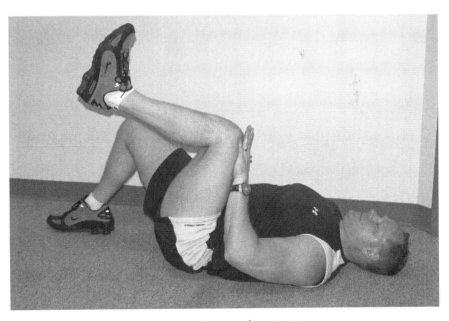

(Psoas Strengthening)

3. **Psoas Release**. Have the person lie on her back, perpendicular to the table so that the legs can hang off. This release is like the *Thomas test* in orthopedics, but we are using it therapeutically (to correct the problem) as well as diagnostically. Make sure the patient is resting his buttocks on the very edge of the table, and then have him lie back, grabbing one knee while you stand very close and hold the down leg. By placing one's self close and holding the leg, the patient will feel a sense of security. This position can make someone fearful of falling since the head is going back while the legs are down and off the table.

Now have the patient attempt to raise the leg that is down and out straight up while you apply resistance. Hold for 5–10 seconds and then release and stretch the leg down. Repeat this stretch three times on each leg. Do not forget to ask, "How is the pain now?" Feeling better? Good! Use numbers like, patient at 7/10 and now in this position it is a 3/10. The body is telling us that the position is correcting the problem, or relieving it.

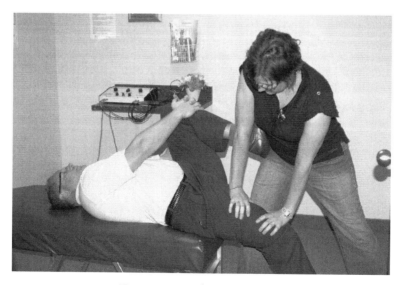

(Psoas Stretch using PNF)

4. **Calf stretch**. A great overall stretch for just about any condition from headaches to low-back, and of course, knee pain. Have the patient stand on a slant board, SOT blocks, or a step where the patient's calves can drop down to stretch. Stay on the slant until the calves feel even and loose. Some people may be so tight that they fall backward, so position the patient close to a wall for support. Again, is it making the person better?

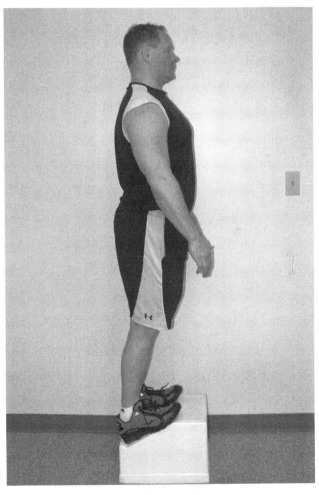

(Calf Stretch)

CHAPTER NINETEEN

TROUBLESHOOTING

Occasionally, I have a patient who does not respond to treatment, which, I confess, stumps me. When this occurs, I carefully review the patient's complaints, my assessment, and the work we've done. After going through this process, I usually discover there are a few obstacles at work to block the patient's healing process, which I then systematically try to eliminate.

One obstacle is ineffective communication with the patient. The patient might be focused on looking for pain, as was the case with an athlete who complained of extreme low-back pain. He exercised and stretched, but when I asked about his pain, he would say, "The pain is still there." Initially, I thought he meant that the pain did not change. I was stumped until I realized that I was not asking the right question. By rephrasing my questions and asking for more detailed responses, I learned that his pain had been reduced by 50 percent. Once I had the patient quantify the stimulus, I soon realized what to do to alleviate his pain. Additionally, I learned that this patient was focused on his pain, as opposed to seeking a solution to alleviate it. If the mind seeks problems, it will find problems. If the mind seeks solutions, guess what? It will find solutions.

The second obstacle is that I overthink the problem rather than listen to the patient and observe his movements. Occasionally, I go into the exam room with a preconceived notion about what is wrong and how to remedy it. Those preconceived notions limit my scope of the *big picture*. If I go into the exam room thinking the patient's problem is in the knee, then I might not observe the patient's problem with the hip, the opposite ankle, generalized posture, and generalized body movements. I also filter out all other data the patient says about his overall health. When this occurs, I must remember to take in the whole picture and not limit my visual and mental focus. Sometimes it becomes necessary to take a step back, or even reschedule the patient's office visit because it is critically important at all times to be totally focused on the patient when making a diagnosis and beginning treatment.

The third obstacle is the patient himself because he has no real awareness of himself or his body. His analytical mind is in *overdrive* and he does not trust what I'm doing to help him or his body's response to it. When this occurs, I work carefully to establish trust and build rapport. It is necessary for the patient to find his own comfort level so that we can address and alleviate his physical complaints.

Here is another scenario I run into: a patient is doing well and then suddenly he is not. We do all the things that usually work for him, but he still does not improve. Why is this? Some people have a hidden motivator; they actually feel guilty about feeling good or feeling better, sometimes because they receive attention only when they are ill or in pain. They substitute attention for love. Others have been trained to believe they do not deserve to enjoy a feeling of wellness or happiness. Instead, they believe they need to be punished, and pain is a way to serve that punishment. This self-destructive behavior must be corrected before the patient can be made whole.

I know this is starting to sound like a psychology lesson, but the mind and body are connected. A patient who is caught up in this pattern may need additional help from an NLP therapist, a psychologist, or other mental health expert. Another, more subtle method might be to suggest a book like, *The Sedona Method,* by Hale Dwoskin, or the use of emotional freedom technique (EFT).

Again, this is about letting go so the healing process may begin. Some people have a hard time letting go of their pain because their whole life has been based around being in pain. Why? Because being in pain gave them something to talk about and use to gain attention. Be very careful not to get caught up in the patient's self-destructive cycle.

This is not meant to be cruel. I am simply providing information for your consideration the next time you have a patient who does not respond to care. It is in the patient's best interest that you refer him or her to a specialist.

There is a save technique for these people—humor. Make them laugh and distract them from their troubles. The mind is like a computer; if the bad program is interrupted, the computer will reset. Keep changing the subject and tell stories about a wonderful vacation or a patient who is doing well. Only give attention to positive things like getting better. That is if you choose to keep the patient.

The most common obstacle I have encountered in a patient who is not responding to care is fear. Some patients are just plain afraid. They are afraid of us and afraid of the pain. Until the patient trusts us, it will be difficult to find out what is wrong. That is right; we will not be able to employ the *getting better or getting worse* method of stimulus introductions. Why? The patient's mind is set up so that we do not hurt him. His primary goal is to leave the office feeling no worse than when he came in. The result is he will not get hurt, but he will not get better, either.

There is a lot of psychology or soul-searching in this chapter but the mind and body are connected and a failure to address both often gives inconsistent results. Dr. Mawell Matlz wrote a book called *Psychocybernetics* that can expound on some of these concepts.

One concept is that our minds, much like a computer, just run programs; therefore, if the program (goal) is set to *not get hurt*, then this is the most likely outcome. A patient who is afraid will not allow us to help him. Without setting a proper goal and moving past fear, the patient will not respond to treatment. Get the patient to tell you what his goal is for his health. Not your goal—the patient's goal. Make the patient describe it in vivid detail because the greater the detail, the more specific the destination.

In addition, the patient's will is the *mental muscle* that makes things happen. If the patient is strong-willed, he is likely to resist any treatment that he does not understand. Again, humor works well to soften a strong-willed patient, and when the opportunity presents itself come beside him. Coming beside a patient and standing by him is a tool that lets the patient know that you are on his side. Standing across from someone is an adversarial position, like two football teams, or soldiers on a battlefield. Each side stands against the other.

As you gain the patient's trust, do simple little things that reassure her that you are there to help and what you are doing is not painful. Secondly, take the time to explain what you are doing and why, before you do it. Show the patient first and move very slowly. Fast movements just create more agitation in the patient because you are moving too fast, or way ahead of them.

226

As human beings we have a primal animal quality. Dealing with a human for the first time can be like dealing with a dog because, in fact, some human responses are similar to canine responses. If we approach a dog too quickly, some dogs will run away, some will bark, some will let you pet them, others will growl and turn on you. Dealing with patients is not much different. Some will let you help them, some will be defensive, some will be adversarial or aggressive, and some will run away. If you have ever watched the TV show, *The Dog Whisperer* with Cesar Milan, you can see what I mean. You can learn a lot about being a better doctor just by viewing this particular show.

Since we are talking about the psyche or soul, we also need to talk about stress. Why? Well, because stress is thought to cause 90% of all disease. If one really looks at a patient's overall health picture, one will see that as a person's stress goes up, so does her pain and health problems. As healers, for us to help our patients or help ourselves, we have to address certain thought processes. *Stinking thinking leads to stinking problems and stinking results.* It is a known fact the brain learns by repetition, and repetition of bad thoughts translates into somatic and organic pains. The body, in my opinion, is a replication of the mind.

The method of *Miracles in Minutes* is to find any or all things that improve life or replicate life. Stress is not life. A plant does not worry about growing up and neither should man. A plant does not feel bad about showing its flower and neither should we feel bad about being ourselves. Stand tall, because life does the same thing.

Another unique method is eye tracking. You can have the patient track your finger or his finger. If any eye movement creates stress or an uncomfortable feeling, have the patient stare at your finger or his and hold the position until the uncomfortable feeling goes away. The eyes are like the mouse on your computer. By holding the eyes in a certain position the brain can, sort of, *rewire* any emotion it has.

Another technique that deals extremely well with stress is NLP, which is a study of human excellence. Things happen in our mind before they happen in our body. Ask anyone who has had a nightmare and soon he or she realizes that nothing was really happening except thought patterns; however, the body did pant, the palms did get clammy, and a person might even sweat. What was he doing? In reality, just sleeping.

I know NLP is controversial, but I have seen it work. Again, do an Internet search to learn more about it or something called, *Time Line Therapy*. I am not an expert on this subject but I can tell you this stuff is powerful. Many major businesses use NLP to improve sales or improve their work force. Why? It works with a high degree of predictability and the results are often spectacular.

We have covered stress and the ramifications of how stress can interfere with healing or progress. In dealing with the general public there are all kinds of people and some of those people create unique challenges to the care givers. At times we run into patients that just seem like they want to argue as one is attempting to help them. Some patients have been conditioned to have something called a fixed mindset. A fixed mindset is when someone is resistant to change and learning new things, i.e. the mind is fixed vs. being open. Carol S. Dweck, PhD., has written a book called *Mindset* subtitle *The New Psychology of Success*. It is a great read on understanding human behavior and possibly helping patients open up to new possibilities and methods of care.

Now if it is none of the above, issues of mental stress or mindsets that are preventing forward progress, then we need to look at how the method is being applied.

1. Are you holding the person in a position until the pain is almost gone or is reduced by 50%? If no, then do this.
2. Are you hesitant or confused? Hesitation is fear, and people can feel your fear thus confidence does not move across the table. Practice the exercises on yourself or family member and see if it produces the light, tall, energy, feel-good sensations indicating that we are moving towards life.
3. Maybe you are doing too much or too many exercises. Pick one or two and stick with it or back down the time and intensity of the exercise. Sometimes less is more.
4. Maybe the person needs a brace. Brace and see.
5. Maybe you are overthinking it. Step back from it and take a deep breath. Now whatever you were doing before now do the opposite or look at the opposite side of the body or opposite direction like south (lower back) or north (neck).
6. Did we check the numbers, or the VAS scale of 0–10 before doing anything?
7. Did we check the numbers 10 seconds into the exercise?
8. Are we looking for the 20% effort and 80% return or are we just "exercising" because "Dr. Wood told me to"?
9. Are we assuming "we know" already? "I said hip pain;" therefore, it has to be the hip. Maybe... maybe not.

What I have found in life is that the answers are usually staring us right in the eye; we are just too blind to see them. That means stop thinking and just be open to anything and especially the unusual. The unusual, or the unexpected are typically where miracles are found, and they can occur in minutes. It is not what you think, but what you know; which is also known as your *gut* or first instinct. Trust that part of your psyche, the *knowing* part, and attempt to truly understand it.

RESEARCH ARTICLES:

J Physiol. 2000 January 1; 522(Pt 1): 165–175.

Activation of the human diaphragm during a repetitive postural task

Paul W Hodges and S C Gandevia

How are the respiratory and 'postural' functions of the diaphragm organised? Our data suggest that diaphragm EMG has three components: increased tonic activity, phasic modulation with respiration and phasic modulation with movement (Fig. 7a). Two questions must be considered regarding the organisation of these components. First, where do the inputs arise from? Secondly, where are they integrated? There are at least four relevant inputs to phrenic motoneurones (Fig. 7b): descending drive from ponto-medullary respiratory centres, drives from non-respiratory supraspinal structures including the motor cortex, spinal interneuronal networks, and inputs from peripheral receptors. The respiratory component of diaphragm activity is derived largely from the respiratory centres (Monteau & Hilaire, 1991). In contrast there are several sources of postural input. For *single* repetitions of voluntary limb movement the perturbation to trunk stability is predictable and is controlled in a feed forward manner (Belen'kii *et al.* 1967; Bouisset & Zattara, 1981;

231

Aruin & Latash, 1995; Hodges & Richardson, 1997; Hodges et al. 1999). This feed forward response recruits the diaphragm (Hodges et al. 1997) and is generated by supraspinal structures (including the cortex, basal ganglia and cerebellum) in parallel with the command for limb movement (Massion, 1992). Correspondingly, there are corticospinal projections to the human diaphragm (Gandevia & Rothwell, 1987) and cortical projections to the medullary respiratory centres (Bassal et al. 1981). The organisation of the postural responses associated with repetitive movement may rely on spinal reflexes, at least for the trunk extensor muscles (Zedka & Prochazka, 1997).

http://www.pubmedcentral.nih.gov/articlerender.fcgi?artid=2269747

J Appl Physiol 103: 48-54, 2007. First published February 15, 2007; doi:10.1152/japplphysiol.00850.2006
8750-7587/07 $8.00

Tonic-to-phasic shift of lumbo-pelvic muscle activity during 8 weeks of bed rest avδ 6-months follow up

Daniel L. Belavý,[1,2,3] **Carolyn A. Richardson,**[2] **Stephen J. Wilson,**[1] **Dieter Felsenberg,**[3] **and Jörn Rittweger**[4]

[1]*School of Information Technology and Electrical Engineering,* [2]*School of Health and Rehabilitation Sciences, The University of Queensland, Brisbane, Australia;* [3]*Zentrum für Muskel-und Knochenforschung, Charité Campus Benjamin Franklin, Berlin, Germany; and* [4]*Institute for Biophysical and Clinical Research into Human Movement, Manchester Metropolitan University, Alsager, Cheshire, United Kingdom*

Submitted 2 August 2006 ; accepted in final form 8 February 2007

Whether changes in proprioceptive function are involved in muscle and motor control change in unloading has been debated by other authors (e.g., 41). The essential suggestion is that the deeper extensor muscles, with a greater density of muscle spindles (36, 38, 56) and slow muscle fiber (24), are more dependent on homonymous afferent input for their normal activity patterns (8, 40, 41). Afferent input has also been shown to be important in the support of tonic muscle activation and activation of slow motor units (7, 8, 47). In unloading, evidence strongly suggests that afferent muscle spindle input decreases (23, 26, 27, 37, 57). This suggests that a reduction in proprioceptive input could underlie the observed shift toward phasic activation patterns in the short lumbar extensors during bed rest and that histochemical fiber type changes may also result.

These neurophysiological studies do not, however, readily explain the effects seen in follow up. After bed rest, the tonic-to-phasic shift appears to accentuate in the extensor muscle systems. Proprioceptive input is normally thought to be restored upon reintroduction of normal gravitational load (16, 23, 26, 27). However, we observed the tonic-to-phasic shift in activation patterns to persist up to 6 months after bed rest in the short lumbar extensors. While this could suggest that normal proprioceptive input was not restored, the underlying mechanisms are unclear.

http://jap.physiology.org/cgi/content/full/103/1/48

J Appl Physiol 101: 1118-1126, 2006. First published June 8, 2006; doi:10.1152/japplphysiol.00165.2006 8750-7587/06 $8.00

Lumbar and cervical erector spinae fatigue elicit compensatory postural responses to assist in maintaining head stability during walking

Justin J. Kavanagh,[1,2,3] Steven Morrison,[1,2] and Rod S. Barrett[1,3]

[1]*School of Physiotherapy and Exercise Science, Griffith Health,* [2]*Applied Cognitive Neuroscience Research Centre, and* [3]*Centre for*

Wireless Monitoring and Applications, Griffith University, Queensland, Australia

Submitted 8 February 2006 ; accepted in final form 31 May 2006

Head stability following fatigue. The results of the present study indicate that walking speed did not differ between any condition. This suggests that not only was the preferred walking speed consistent between control walking trials but that the level of induced LES and CES fatigue did not affect locomotor system's ability to repeat the preferred walking speed. One characteristic of walking often observed with acute and chronic postural deficits is that walking speed is decreased, with a view of minimizing potentially perturbing segmental oscillations, thus enhancing stability. Compared with healthy adults, the elderly (5, 45), Parkinson's disease (40), and cerebral and spinal palsy (7, 21) individuals often exhibit a more cautious walking strategy, which is characterized by adaptations in walking speed and segmental interactions that assist in minimizing the amplitude and variability of head motion. Studying postural control in populations with musculoskeletal degeneration, or any type of coordination deficit, can be problematic due to the cause-and-effect relationship of walking speed and stability. It is often difficult to determine whether adaptations of the neuromuscular system cause reductions in gait speed (22) or whether the slower speed is due to self-imposed constraints to provide a greater perception of stability (20). The absence of speed differences between walking conditions in the present study suggests that differences observed for head stability and segmental attenuation are more likely to reflect the singular effect of fatigue rather than velocity-dependent changes in gait patterns.

http://jap.physiology.org/cgi/content/full/101/4/1118

Balance and Gait in Total Hip Replacement: A Pilot Study.

Research Article

American Journal of Physical Medicine & Rehabilitation. 82(9):669-677, September 2003. *Nallegowda, Mallikarjuna; Singh, U.; Bhan, Surya; Wadhwa, Sanjay; Handa, Gita; Dwivedi, S. N.*

Abstract:

Nallegowda M, Singh U, Bhan S, Wadhwa S, Handa G, Dwivedi SN: Balance and gait in total hip replacement: A pilot study. Am J Phys Med Rehabil 2003;82:669-677.

Objective: Evaluation of balance, gait changes, sexual functions, and activities of daily living in patients with total hip replacement in comparison with healthy subjects.

Design: A total of 30 patients were included in the study after total hip replacement. Balance was examined using dynamic posturography, and gait evaluation was done clinically. Sexual functions and activities of daily living were also assessed. A total of 30 healthy subjects of comparable age and sex served as a control group.

Results: Dynamic balance and gait differed significantly in both the groups. Despite capsulectomy, no significant difference was observed on testing proprioception. In the sensory organization tests with difficult tasks, patients needed more sensory input from vision and vestibular sense, despite normal proprioceptive sense. **Significant difference was observed for limits of stability, rhythmic weight shifts, and for gait variables other than walking base. Some of the patients had major difficulties with sexual functions and activities of daily living.**

Conclusions: Compared with the healthy age- and sex-matched controls, patients with total hip replacement did not have any proprioceptive deficit. Patients required extrasensory input, and there was a delayed motor response. Gait and dynamic balance results also indicated the motor deficit and required a compensatory strategy. Restoration of the postural control in these patients is thus essential. Necessary training is required for balance, gait, and activities of daily living, and proper sexual counseling is necessary in postoperative care.

Abstract

Freeman, Jacklyn Harrell. **Evaluating the Effects of Age on the Variability in Lifting**

Technique.

(Under the direction of Dr. Gary A. Mirka)

1.1.1.1 Muscle strength

It has been documented that aging can lead to progressive decreases in physical

capability, which include decreases in muscle strength, aerobic power, thermoregulation,

reaction speed, and acuity of the ocular and auditory senses (Shepard, 2000). Wright and

Mital (1999) report that muscle strength is a primary measure of physical capacity, and that aging can lead to the gradual reduction in muscle strength capabilities. In their research, they found that these declines in muscle strength can make completing daily activities harder for older individuals. This is shown by the statistic that the percentage of individuals between the ages of 45 and 84 needing assistance in completing daily tasks doubles each succeeding decade.

Okada *et al.* (2001) conducted a study investigating the effects of a sudden deceleration resulting from postural disturbance in eight elderly men (67-72 years) and eight younger men (19-22 years). Even though their study focused on age-related differences in postural control, Okada *et al.* also looked at flexion and extension strength at the ankle and knee joints.

Surface electromyography data was obtained from the anterior tibialis muscle and the medial head of the gastrocnemius muscle of the right leg. Their results indicated that when compared to the younger group, the older subject group had lower muscle forces in their extremities. Dorsal flexion, plantar flexion, knee extension, and knee flexion all were significantly less in the older subject group than in the younger group.

http://www.lib.ncsu.edu/theses/available/etd-05172005-180047/unrestricted/etd.pdf

Made in the USA
San Bernardino, CA
03 June 2013